Palgrave Studies in Literature, Science and Medicine

Palgrave Studies in Literature, Science and Medicine is an exciting, prize-winning series that focuses on one of the most vibrant and interdisciplinary areas in literary studies: the intersection of literature, science and medicine. Comprised of academic monographs, essay collections, and Palgrave Pivot books, the series will emphasize a historical approach to its subjects, in conjunction with a range of other theoretical approaches. The series will cover all aspects of this rich and varied field and is open to new and emerging topics as well as established ones.

Mary Chapman

Writing Women's Madness, 1845–1914

palgrave
macmillan

Mary Chapman
Department of English
University of Liverpool
Liverpool, UK

ISSN 2634-6435 ISSN 2634-6443 (electronic)
Palgrave Studies in Literature, Science and Medicine
ISBN 978-3-031-97091-7 ISBN 978-3-031-97092-4 (eBook)
https://doi.org/10.1007/978-3-031-97092-4

This work was supported by White Rose College of the Arts and Humanities.

Cover credit: whitemay

This Palgrave Macmillan imprint is published by the registered company Springer Nature Switzerland AG
The registered company address is: Gewerbestrasse 11, 6330 Cham, Switzerland

Acknowledgments This book would not have been possible without the generous gift of time, expertise, and support from esteemed friends and colleagues.

I am grateful to Professor James Mussell who, aside from being an excellent doctoral supervisor, encouraged my curiosity about nineteenth-century periodicals and provided guidance and knowledge which has been invaluable to this project. Thanks also, to Dr. Michael A. Finn, without whose expertise in the history of psychiatry I would have been very much astray.

I would like to express my gratitude to Professor Claire Brock and Professor Katy Mullin, who gave such thoughtful and helpful comments on my doctoral thesis, with suggestions for turning the research into this book.

I would also like to thank the staff at Palgrave Macmillan, particularly Molly Beck, whose enthusiasm for the project was encouraging from the start. Thanks also to my anonymous reader, whose feedback was considerate and extremely helpful.

Lastly, I am enormously grateful to my husband, Tom, who supported me throughout the research for this book (including during a hiatus for the birth of our son), and who has always been my loudest cheerleader.

This research was supported by an AHRC Doctoral Studentship from the White Rose College of the Arts & Humanities.

Competing Interests The author han no competing interests to declare that are relevant to the content of this manuscript.

Contents

About the Author

Dr. Mary Chapman is the William Noble Fellow at the University of Liverpool. Dr Chapman's research focuses on the periodical press and medical practice during the Victorian period. Her work centres on women in medicine, as both practitioners and patients. She has published on perceptions of the female mind in the Victorian press (*Victorian Periodicals Review*, 2020), on medical women's magazines (*Humanities*, 2024), and on Amy Levy and melancholia (*Women's Writing*, 2024).

Abbreviations

CRI	Crichton Royal Institution
JMS	*Journal of Mental Science*
LCH	Lady Chichester Hospital
LSMW	London School of Medicine for Women
MPA	Medico-Psychological Association (formerly Association of Medical Officers of Asylums and Hospitals for the Insane)

List of Figures

List of Tables

CHAPTER 1

Introduction: Understanding the Nineteenth-Century Mind Sciences in their Scientific and Cultural Context

Building On a Feminist Historiography

In the nineteenth century, women were understood to be especially vulnerable to insanity on account of their biology. The female reproductive system was thought to have a powerful effect on the nerves, making women's minds unstable and prone to specific kinds of mental disease linked to the activity of the uterus and ovaries. Psychiatrists thus diagnosed and treated women for reproductive as well as mental and behavioural symptoms. This fostered a belief in the gendered mind which was formalised into a coherent hypothesis of female madness by the psychiatric profession. Foundational feminist scholarship, such as the work of Elaine Showalter (1987), Caroll Smith-Rosenberg and Charles Rosenberg (1973), and Sandra Gilbert and Susan Gubar (1979), has demonstrated that nineteenth-century psychiatric theories about the female brain were informed by contemporary cultural beliefs about women, which emphasised their domestic and maternal role in society and were often misogynistic. These scholars have drawn their conclusions from the similarities between such theories and the dominant ideology of gender during this period, in particular the central importance of reproductive biology to both medical and lay beliefs about women's physical and mental capacities. Early psychiatrists viewed the female brain from a

M. Chapman, *Writing Women's Madness, 1845–1914*, Palgrave Studies in Literature, Science and Medicine,
https://doi.org/10.1007/978-3-031-97092-4_1

position of ideological bias, seeing women's minds as inferior for the same reason that women fulfilled an inequal position in society.

Elaine Showalter (1987) has argued that more women than men were found mad in the nineteenth century, in part because of gendered beliefs about the unstable female mind, but also due to the oppressions of patriarchal society, which put an emotional and mental strain on many women, making them more likely to suffer from mental illness. According to Showalter, women who did suffer from insanity were sick because of the strict constraints imposed upon them by society, either because they broke down under them or rebelled against the 'concepts of normality and deviance that women perforce must accept' (Showalter 1987, p. 20). Phyllis Chesler (2005) has likewise offered a radical perspective on female insanity, arguing that women were found mad simply because their behaviour did not fit within the boundaries of social acceptability in Victorian society. Chesler states that 'most women in asylums were not insane' (Chesler 2005, p. 62), and that women were punished for 'either acting out of the devalued female role or the total or partial rejection of one's sex role stereotype' (Chesler 2005, p. 116). Chesler argues that proper adherence to social expectations was an important measure of mental health in women, whilst character traits perceived as unfeminine, such as 'physical aggression, grandeur, sexuality and emotionality' were markers of madness (Chesler 2005, p. 91). Similarly, Denise Russell has argued that the expansion of medical discourse into the study of the mind turned 'many moral categories into medical ones. What in the past had been wrong came to be seen as diseased or unhealthy' (Russell 1995, p. 12). The psychiatric profession therefore 'appropriated the social right to pass judgement' about female morality, exerting a 'corrective force' through incarcerating women in asylums (Russell 1995, p. 12).

These studies rightly highlight the important role social and cultural beliefs had to play in the theory and treatment of female insanity during the nineteenth century. Yet the larger claims about the oppressive nature of psychiatry which these formative studies made have been contested by more recent quantitative historiography on diagnostic patterns and patient populations in Victorian asylums. These studies refute the idea of a controlling profession, intent on suppressing vulnerable women. Jonathan Andrews and Anne Digby (2004) have edited a useful volume of essays on gender and class in the treatment of mental illness. They suggest that 'within the asylum women occupied more complex roles than the earlier stereotype of powerless victims subdued by arbitrary diagnoses' (Andrews and Digby 2004, p. 30). Arguing that ‘as a microcosm of society’ the asylum reflected ‘ordinary values and standards of behaviour,’ they do not devalue the usefulness of a gendered analysis but suggest that its value comes from a synthesis of gender and other factors, such as class or ethnicity (Andrews and Digby 2004, p. 30).

It is also clear that patient identity was not the only consideration in the psychiatric treatment of women during the Victorian period. David Wright’s (2004) study of Buckinghamshire Lunatic Asylum demonstrates that hardly any female patients were classified upon admission under disease headings that would denote a specifically gendered aetiology such as hysteria or puerperal mania. He argues that institutional and familial dynamics were more important in decisions made about the confinement of female patients, than gendered theories. Anne Shepard, in her study of two Surrey asylums, contends that whilst doctors did believe ‘women to be more prone to mental disorder,’ any occasional increases in female admissions ‘can be explained by localised factors’ (Shepard 2004, p. 243). Shepard notes that the most significant difference between men and women lay in the residual patients; more women than men remained in the asylum, in both public and private institutions. She suggests that this may have been because, for ‘certain groups of women, life in the asylum was preferable’ to the social isolation of spinsterhood, or ‘the rigours of extended child-bearing and dangerous employment’ (Shepard 2004, p. 243). From these studies, gender emerges as one of several factors relevant to nineteenth-century psychiatric treatment, comparable to its importance in everyday life during this period.

Yet this scholarship, in paying attention to the quotidian detail of actual psychiatric practice, has not investigated how such practices fit alongside shifting medical ideas about the female mind. Further research is needed to discover how the different factors which these studies detail (from treatment methodologies to class-specific institutional management practices) dovetail with mind doctors’ beliefs about their patients. This is necessary to understand how the social and cultural values held by clinical practitioners influenced and were supported by the scientific methodologies and administrative practices of their discipline. Conversely, the social control model of early feminist historians, whilst excellent in unearthing the ideological basis of theories of female madness, ignores several significant factors in the development of psychiatry in the nineteenth century. For example, the evolution of expertise; changing scientific beliefs about appropriate and effective treatments; and the expansion of professional activities outside of the asylum, through education, literature and medical societies. Nineteenth-century theories of female insanity were not merely ideology applied to the treatment of mad women but were conceived through the influence of shifting epistemologies of the mind, brain and nervous system, as well as the methodologies of clinical practice which developed with the professionalisation of medical care for the insane.

It was during the nineteenth century that a shift from a spiritual to a physiological model of the mind occurred. This strengthened the authority of the physician in treating madness. The asylum became the predominant site for the administration of medical care for the insane, moving the responsibility for the mad from the community to the institution, and emphasising the doctor's expertise. As treatment for insanity incorporated a medical understanding of the mind, those working in the field needed to throw out their old methods and put forward new theories that fitted within the disease model of madness. Gendered theories of the female mind, based in reproductive biology, were made possible by the development of this new medical attitude to insanity which placed the human mind within a physiological framework. The development of psychiatry as a profession was therefore just as integral to the shaping of theories of female insanity, as cultural notions of femininity.

This book builds upon the historiography of female madness to present a holistic analysis of the psychiatric treatment of women in the nineteenth century, one which examines gendered beliefs about the female mind within the clinical context of the emerging profession. Explaining the connection between gendered ideologies and theories of female madness as simply the prejudices of mind doctors tells us little about the ways in which these medical concepts were formed. Previous scholarship has yet to demonstrate how cultural and medical discourses were connected and explain the transference of ideas between them. This transference has been taken for granted as an inevitable consequence of patriarchal Victorian society, a supposition that ignores the active process of transformation that must necessarily have taken place for cultural ideas to be applied in a clinical setting. If we are to gain a better understanding of psychiatric theories of the female brain, we therefore need to place these theories within the wider intellectual context of the developing mind sciences.

This context is important, not only because it shaped the contemporary concept of insanity and therefore what beliefs about the female mind were possible, but because it influenced the way in which ideas were produced and communicated within the profession. Written discourse was one of the primary ways in which psychiatry established itself as a legitimate field of medicine, whether through medical journals and other scholarly publications, or the documents of clinical practice such as case notes and annual reports. New theories were formulated, communicated and consolidated through writing. As a result, texts are the main site where we can see the development of gendered medical beliefs in action, the needs of the developing profession shaping where and how knowledge was articulated. Ideas about female insanity were formed through and by writing during this period.

This book will explore how the process of discipline formation impacted the development of gendered ideas within the psychiatric profession, and how this was expressed through writing. In doing so, this book places nineteenth-century medical beliefs about the female mind in their full historical context and critically analyses the mechanisms through which they were created. The unique circumstances of an establishing medical specialty encouraged the reconstruction of social ideology as medical fact, which was then transformed into clinical reality through texts essential to psychiatric practice. This book focuses on two areas of written discourse that were the principal instrument of communication, professionalisation and knowledge transfer in psychiatry during this period: clinical literature and periodicals. Clinical texts such as textbooks, case notes and institutional records shaped the development of gendered theories by organising patient information within specific narratives. In contrast, periodicals allowed for these theories to be adapted and contested by sharing knowledge about the female mind within and beyond the profession. This book discusses the textuality of these sources, exploring how their genre, form, language and readership shaped beliefs about women's brains. These textual features, and the ideas they communicated, were shaped by the needs of the developing profession.

This research thus brings together studies of Victorian attitudes towards the female mind with historical accounts of the professionalisation of the medical treatment of insanity. This latter body of work includes studies by historians such as Andrew Scull (1993), Edward Shorter (1998), and Michel Foucault (1999), and describes how care of the mad shifted from the community to the institution over the nineteenth century. These historians have argued that the theory and practice of psychiatry during this period was motivated by doctors' desire to establish recognition for the new discipline and retain jurisdiction over the mentally ill at a time when medicine had little to offer in the way of cures for insanity. This chapter will therefore first review the development of psychiatric medicine, which provides important background for this current study, and is the historiographical foundation on which this research has been built.[1]

The Changing Paradigm of Madness

Key to any investigation of how gendered theories of the female mind were formed, is an understanding of the intellectual context in which these ideas developed. In particular, the move towards a medical concept of insanity during the first half of the nineteenth century was fundamental in establishing the primacy of reproductive biology in theories of women's madness. Prior to the Enlightenment, insanity was commonly understood within a religious framework. Lunacy was a bestial state caused by the loss of the eternal soul through sin or demonic possession. However, in the eighteenth century, the insane began to be viewed as human beings who had instead undergone a loss of reason. It was in this context that the study of the mind gradually shifted from a philosophical to a physiological discipline, and the concept of insanity as an illness became possible.

In the early 1800s, the mind was beginning to be understood as the seat of thought and action within the body, believed to be proof of humanity's pre-eminence in the chain of being (Smith 2004, 1997). Rick Rylance has shown how a 'Christian conception of humanity' stressed the special status of humans, who held exclusive spiritual rights in the natural kingdom (Rylance 2000, p. 24). Mankind occupied an important place 'at the pinnacle of Creation' and the marvellous abilities of the human mind were fitted for this purpose, representing the wonderful design of God in nature (Rylance 2000, p. 25). As a result, 'psychologically, human beings were thought to possess relatively autonomous, distinctively human, mental *faculties*' (Rylance 2000, p. 27). However, the emphasis on man's connection with God meant that the powers of the human mind were believed to be 'entirely determined' by the spirit, and the body and spirit were 'ontologically distinct' (Rylance 2000, p. 23). Psychology, 'functionally as well as etymologically,' meant simply '"the study of the soul"' (Rylance 2000, p. 22).

[1] For a full discussion of how this research engages with studies in the history of psychiatry more broadly, see the conclusion to this book (Chapter 6).

Robert M. Young has described how the Christian concept of human psychology defined the mind and body 'in such a way that any relationship between them seemed impossible' (Young 1968, p. 252). Whilst the body was 'matter, [...] passive, and law-like,' the mind was 'active, and free' (Young 1968, p. 252). Despite this, human experience demonstrated that the spiritual mind clearly interacted with the physical flesh. The task of science was to understand how 'impressions on the sense organs caused ideas, and thoughts caused movements,' despite this process being apparently inconceivable (Young 1968, p. 252). Inheriting this concept of the metaphysical mind, early nineteenth-century philosophers approached the problem from a Cartesian perspective, reasoning that there existed a dualism of mind and body: two distinct systems, operating sympathetically. The idea that humans possessed mental functions separate from their physical body led to the emergence of the school of faculty psychology during the first decades of the nineteenth century. In this school, human mental faculties were arranged hierarchically, with the higher faculties such as reason, faith, love and the exercise of the will placed above the lower faculties like sensation, feeling, appetite and desire. This division clearly placed the different functions of the brain along a psychological-physiological divide, attributing greater value to the faculties which seemed to express the essence of the human soul (Rylance 2000).

The question remained, however, as to how these dual systems of mind and body were connected. German neuroanatomist and physiologist Franz Joseph Gall attempted to answer this question in what Young terms the 'first empirical approach' to faculty psychology (Young 1968, p. 253). Gall developed a theory of cerebral localisation, isolating the faculties in different parts of the brain. Later known as phrenology, his work established the idea that 'the brain is the organ of the mind' and implied the revolutionary concept that 'psychology is not a branch of epistemology, but of general biology' (Young 1968, p. 254). Although Gall's phrenology was later refuted, he played a crucial role in instituting a physiological approach within the field and catalysed further study. In the 1820s and 30s Johannes Müller and Charles Bell established the sensory-motor link between the brain and body. They identified the cortex as the distinct area of the brain which they believed to house the mind and will. This was separate from the lower centres of the organ, which controlled movement and other bodily functions through the nervous system. Their study explained how the mind (including the higher faculties it exhibited) and physiological sensations (the lower faculties) were connected to the brain. The supporters of this version of faculty psychology thus attempted to empirically confirm the assumptions made by eighteenth-century natural theologians, arguing that although the mind worked through the body, it remained a separate entity (Rylance 2000; Young 1968).

However, by the middle of the nineteenth century faculty psychology had its detractors. Jenny Bourne Taylor (2010) has demonstrated how an opposing philosophy of mind had fostered a different approach to psychology, which attempted to explain the mind–body connection using an input model. Known as associationist psychology, the theory originated in the philosophy of John Locke, who had argued for a concept of mind in which 'consciousness derived from experience' (Bourne Taylor 2010, p. 185). These ideas were given a physiological rationale by David Hartley in the eighteenth century, which was adopted by the associationist school. This school proposed that the 'structures of the mind were formed by sensory and perceptual stimulation,' with ideas being created through sequence or contiguity (Rylance 2000, p. 57). In the 1850s and 60s, respected psychologists such as William Carpenter, Alexander Bain and G. H. Lewes all 'combined associationism and sensory-motor physiology' in their work 'to analyse the connections as well as the gradations between reflex, habit, instinct, emotion and thought' (Bourne Taylor 2010, p. 195). The brain, its distinct regions, and the role of the nervous system were all acknowledged as fundamental to understanding the embodied mind. Although the human will remained a separate faculty, it was perceived as interconnected to the physiological functions of the brain, which were influenced by external factors, such as lived experience, and produced psychological results, such as memories. Whilst associationist psychology maintained that the mind and body were distinct, the theory placed them in closer connection than faculty psychology and attempted to explain the functional and structural detail of the link between them.

As the century progressed, the dualistic model of the mind and body became more complex. Advancements in technology and instrumentation fostered the growth of psychophysiology, as it became possible to put forward scientific findings from experimental laboratory work. These experiments built on the work of the associationist school and focused on the role of the sensory-motor arc in linking the brain to the nervous system, as well as the function of different parts of the anatomy of the brain. A more detailed understanding of cerebral localisation was possible after the work of David Ferrier, for example, who demonstrated that specific areas of the brain controlled motor function (Star 1989). Herbert Spencer was also influential in his application of theories of evolution to the human psyche; the structure of which he believed to mirror species development from simple to complex forms. A variety of different explanations were suggested for many aspects of human mental life.

These diverse theories about the brain shared a physiological framework but they also maintained the perceived interconnection between the mind and body which necessarily implied that the two were separate entities; a position strengthened by John Hughlings Jackson's work on the nervous system. Roger Smith argues that theological and philosophical conceptions of the human mind continued to influence the science that was being done and the conclusions that were being drawn from it; 'the basic terms and framework for discussion of mind and brain came from religious and moral preoccupations' (Smith 2004, p. 84). It was the adherence to Christian beliefs about man's relationship to the divine that limited and directed developing hypotheses and ensured the continued support of a separate, but linked, metaphysical mind and physical brain. Smith suggests that this concept of selfhood had such 'absolute centrality' to the epistemological basis for being human, that it was enshrined as necessarily core to any medical or scientific theory made (Smith 2004, p. 96). Despite the obvious danger of accusations of materialism in physiological psychology, Victorian scientists argued that the more they discovered about the mind, the more it proved the existence of the human self, or soul.

It was alongside these developments in the science of the human mind that attitudes towards disturbances of mind shifted. Although psychology did not deal with mental disease, it provided an epistemological basis for mental health care as the development of the mind-brain connection made psychological medicine conceivable. The changing psychological paradigm was crucial in placing madness within a medical context: if the mind was connected to physiological processes, insanity could be viewed as a physical rather than spiritual disease, and a secular and medical response was therefore necessary. The theoretical framework for insanity was also founded on the dualism of mind and body that was the key tenet of the psychological sciences and included a belief in the agency of a separate human will. Michael J. Clark (1981) has shown how Victorian physicians believed that madness was caused by a *physiological* change which resulted in negative psychological manifestations such as delusions or altered emotional states. In the mentally ill, the 'normal [...] autonomy of psychical life was severely reduced' and 'thought and feeling were progressively removed from the sphere of volitional control' (Clark 1981, p. 275). This loss of will was believed to be caused by 'diseased physical processes' that 'spilled over' from the physical organism into what, in the healthy person, would have been the 'separate and closed domain of the mind' (Clark 1981, p. 276). Insanity was therefore seen as a 'disorder of the mind resulting from a structural or functional lesion of the "organ of the mind," the brain' (Clark 1981, p. 276). The nerves and other organs of the body could also have a role to play in this process, factors which, we shall see, assumed an even greater significance in discussions of female mental health.

Significantly, a physiological model of madness increased potential for cure and placed the doctor (instead of the priest) in the role of caregiver for the mentally ill. The idea that insanity was a bodily disease which could (and should) be treated meant that mentally ill people began to be viewed as patients. This facilitated the rise of psychiatry as a profession. In England, this shift occurred primarily through the institutions that housed the insane population. Prior to the early 1800s, specific provision for the mentally ill was made by the community through charitable hospitals such as Bethlem, or—for those who could afford to pay the fees—small private asylums, or madhouses. More often, the mad were the problem of the workhouses to deal with as they saw fit. Andrew Scull has argued that madness was not generally viewed as a 'socially significant' form of deviance and the insane were therefore housed (if at all) in institutions devoted to an 'amorphous mass' of the 'indigent, troublesome, and morally disreputable' (Scull 1979, p. 36). However, 'emerging at the end of the eighteenth century' alongside changing beliefs about the nature of madness 'was a growing market or trade in lunacy' which Scull terms 'the breeding ground' for professionalisation in the medical care of the insane (Scull 1979, p. 43). A growing recognition of abuses and appalling treatment within these private houses, which were often operated for profit and whose proprietors were little concerned with the health of their inmates, led to a reform movement that instigated the growth of a state-run network of asylums in England.

Beginning with an 1807 investigation into York Asylum, this movement was spearheaded by middle-class philanthropists, who saw the current state of asylums as an affront to their Evangelical values of humanitarianism and paternalism and believed that the chaos inherent in the haphazard network of institutions was a hindrance to social progress (Brown 2006). These campaigners pushed for a centralised, state-controlled administration of mental health care which would both protect lunatic patients and prevent them from becoming a danger to the community. The reformers undertook a series of investigations into the conditions at various asylums around the country, producing several Select Committee reports on the horrible brutalities they witnessed. These calls to reform resulted in a series of legislative moves during the first four decades of the nineteenth century, culminating in the reform of lunacy law in 1845. This legislation was split into two interdependent bills: the County Asylums Act and Lunacy Act, passed on 4th and 8th August of that year. The former required each county to establish an asylum for the reception of pauper lunatics and the latter made regular external inspection of all asylums by a national Lunacy Commission mandatory. The Acts therefore consolidated and officially recognised a turn towards coordinated institutional care for the insane in England (and Wales; Scotland was not to pass similar legislation until 1857); part of a growing support for state provision for the needy of all kinds. By mid-century, the asylum was therefore an important part of the professional landscape of psychiatry. Therapeutically and legislatively, these institutions had become the recognised space for the housing and treatment of the insane (Scull 1993; Shorter 1998; Arieno 1989).

Treatment of the mad had also changed significantly during this period, as the reformist supervisors of the new asylums sought to replace the old physically coercive model of patient management with a system which was both non-violent and therapeutic. Now that insanity was understood as an illness, it was important that patient behaviour was changed, rather than simply controlled. Moral treatment, pioneered by William Tuke at the York Retreat in the early 1800s, was crucially important to the reform movement as it demonstrated the possibility for managing madness in a peaceful way. The treatment emphasised the removal of mechanical restraint, common in the eighteenth century, and instituted a quasi-medical and professional methodology that involved close care between the physician and patient, with the physician using his personal authority instead of physical beatings to curb irrational behaviour. The intent was to transform the lunatic into a healthy individual once again through focus on the psychology of the patient (Digby 1985, 2004; Glover 1984; Charland 2007). As Scull describes, 'from its architecture to its domestic arrangements, the Retreat was designed to encourage the individual's own efforts to reassert his powers of self-control' over his unreasonable mind (Scull 1979, p. 68). The superintendents of the reformed asylums needed to be qualified to implement such delicate therapies. With the new understanding of the physiological origins of madness, the physician therefore came to be recognised as the rightful authority to be placed at the head of the asylum. Men like John Conolly, resident physician at Middlesex County Asylum from 1839 and famous for popularising the principle of non-restraint, became known as specialists in the field: mind doctors, or alienists.

By mid-century, the medical approach to caring for the insane had developed to focus on physical treatments, reflecting the interest in the nervous system within the mind sciences. Clark has shown that the 'medical treatment of insanity' generally consisted of the attempted 'restoration of the normal functioning' of the organs and nerves perceived to be causing the mental imbalance (Clark 1981, p. 278). He argues that 'leading alienists emphatically rejected' psychotherapeutics, in part because the strategies available, such as hypnotherapy, induced the patient to fall into a state so much like the pathological one they were trying to cure (Clark 1981, p. 278). Despite Clark's claim, there is much evidence to suggest that although physicians adhered to the physiological basis of insanity in theory, the lack of any proven clinical methodologies in the field meant they were willing to try a range of treatments in the hope that the patient would get better: drugs, warm or cold baths, the rest cure, occupational therapy, the physician–patient relationship, and surgery were all used to try to cure mental disease. Nevertheless, madness and its treatments were firmly under medical jurisdiction. By the 1850s, the asylum was seen as a therapeutic institution and those who worked there, caring for the mad, were increasingly placed in the role of medical professional.

The second half of the nineteenth century saw the development of psychiatry as a distinct discipline, with its own professional structures that mirrored those of medicine proper (Porter 1987, 2003; Bynum et al. 2004). In 1841, the Medico-Psychological Association was established for those who worked in the field (originally named the Association of Medical Officers of Asylums and Hospitals for the Insane) and from 1858 the organisation produced its own medical journal, the *Journal of*

Mental Science. Members contributed scholarly articles to the periodical and those at the top of their profession wrote treatises and other scientific publications on the clinical treatment of mental disease. From the 1880s, the profession became more focused on the pathology of insanity and laboratories were set up in asylums such as Claybury in London to run experiments and conduct post-mortem examinations on patients (Clark 1981).

The discipline was not without its problems, however. Formal education in the mind sciences remained extremely limited until the early twentieth century, as psychiatry was still stigmatised as a less prestigious and important branch of medical science. Alienists tended to qualify as MDs before later choosing an asylum role, gaining experience in mental disease either on the job or through the limited number of courses given to medical schools on a visiting basis by senior doctors in the field. In addition, the failure of psychiatry to provide any real or definite cures for a large percentage of the lunatic population led to overcrowding in late-Victorian asylums. Once committed, many patients spent the rest of their lives in institutions and the size of county asylums grew unremittingly. The intellectual climate of the latter decades of the century, with its pessimistic focus on evolutionary regression, also discouraged hope by cultivating a view of madness as irreversible mental degeneration (Scull 1979, 1993; Bartlett and Wright 1999).

Despite the lack of scientific and clinical progress in the field, psychiatry was well established by the early 1900s. Boundaries of practice had been shaped through the growth of the asylum network which provided an institutional space for the profession's activities and encouraged a methodological and therapeutic approach to clinical practice. The professional authority of the practitioners who worked within these spaces was reinforced through legislative action and through disciplinary building activities like scholarly publication which gave the community legitimacy as a medical body. This was strengthened through the eventual introduction of mental disease onto the medical curriculum and certification in the field at the turn of the century. The medical understanding, care and treatment of disturbances of mind at the end of the Victorian period looked very different to the religious philosophies of a hundred years previous.

The Reproductive Basis for Female Insanity and Victorian Ideologies of Gender

The new physiological approach to madness was integral to the development of theories of female insanity during the Victorian period. The concept of insanity as a disease of the body rather than the spirit encouraged mind doctors to look for causes of mental disturbance in pathological changes within the brain, nerves and other organs. In women, the obvious differences of reproductive biology—which appeared so significant in comparison with the male body (considered the default human form)—were thought to be central to the aetiology of mental disease. Elaine Showalter has shown that mind doctors believed the 'instability' of the female reproductive system 'interfered with [women's] sexual, emotional and rational control' (Showalter 1987, p. 55). Inheriting centuries old myths of the wandering uterus and the mysterious and dangerous reproductive organs (Small 1998; Shuttleworth 1996; Ussher 2011), nineteenth-century mind doctors medicalised this lore into a coherent hypothesis of disease. Physicians called this hypothesis '"reflex insanity in women",' referring to the 'connection between the female reproductive and nervous systems' which allowed the uterus and ovaries to influence the function of the brain (Showalter 1987, p. 55).

Reproduction was considered to be woman's most important physiological function and as such reproductive processes had absolute primacy in women's physical and mental health, with every aspect of female biology subservient to this one function. In psychiatry, mind doctors theorised that the uterus and ovaries, connected to the brain through the nervous system, could cause irritation that resulted in disturbances of mind. Conversely, insanity originating from other causes could adversely impact the reproductive system via the nerves, causing physiological problems such as arrested menstruation. This was believed to be because of the intimate sympathy between the reproductive organs and the nervous system and the powerful tax of nervous energy which these organs exerted (Malane 2005; Appignanesi 2009). Cynthia Eagle Russett (1989) has demonstrated how the principle of the conservation of energy, or the First Law of Thermodynamics, was vital in establishing theories of nerve force and women's limited supply of it. The law stated that 'the energy of a system remains always constant, although its usefulness for work may diminish, because energy can neither be created nor destroyed' (Eagle Russett 1989, p. 106). In other words, there was a finite amount of energy in the universe, and it must be carefully maintained. In psychiatry, this translated into 'a theory of mental health defined as the prudential conservation of nerve force' (Eagle Russett 1989, p. 112). Nervous exhaustion could result if care was not taken to monitor one's own nervous supply. In women, this was particularly important for they 'added a singular expense of their own' to the bodily economy: the 'development and maintenance of a highly complex reproductive system' (Eagle Russett 1989, p. 116). The female mind was thus influenced by the ebb and flow of nervous force as the uterus and ovaries required more or less energy at different times in a woman's reproductive life.

Consequently, whenever a woman showed signs of mental disease, physiological changes in her reproductive system were suspected and symptoms related to these organs were considered pertinent. The cessation of menstruation at menopause, for example, was thought to cause a decline in the mental faculties and an increase in emotional instability. Although reproductive biology was considered significant in the diagnosis and treatment of any form of madness in women, the biological basis for female insanity also gave rise to specifically feminine mental illnesses which were thought to be catalysed by the reproductively significant periods of a woman's life. Victims of the periodicity of their bodies, women were believed to be especially vulnerable to insanity during times of change as the activity of the reproductive organs drew a larger amount of energy from their nervous system. Women were also thought to have frailer nervous systems than men and this double jeopardy of aggressive reproductive organs and fragile nerves rendered disease particularly likely. Categories of illness were theorised around female reproduction, including lactational insanity, insanity of puberty (at the onset of menstruation), climacteric insanity (at the onset of menopause), and puerperal insanity (insanity of childbirth). Hysteria was also considered a female disease, thought to be the result of sexual impulses caused by the disturbing influence of the reproductive organs. These diagnoses reflected a belief in the pathology of reproduction and the unstable influence of the uterus and ovaries on women's minds.

For example, Hilary Marland's formative work on puerperal insanity has explored the illness's relationship to 'women's intrinsic biological weakness' (Marland 2004, p. 3). The disease usually appeared 'shortly after childbirth' when women were thought to be 'mentally susceptible' and 'encompassed relatively brief attacks, nervous upsets, violence or delusions, as well as long-term manifestations of mania or deep and protracted melancholia' (Marland 2004, p. 3). Occurring as a direct consequence of reproduction, it was a disease which epitomised Victorian conceptions of woman as 'a victim of her fragile nervous system' and tapped into fears about what lurked beneath the surface of feminine moral control (Marland 2004, p. 6). In disorders that did not exclusively affect women, the suffering of female patients was still interpreted differently to that of their male counterparts. Neurasthenia was a disease which could strike members of both sexes, though it was symbolically feminised. Janet Oppenheim has shown how the disorder was thought to result from 'the pace of contemporary life' and was associated with that 'extremely fragile creature,' the middle-class wife or daughter (Oppenheim 1991, p. 206). The refined woman's great 'liability to nervous illness' rendered her vulnerable to psychic shocks that resulted in exhaustion, exhibited through symptoms such as listlessness, bodily aches and pains, weakness and melancholia (Oppenheim 1991, p. 206). Neurasthenia was therefore associated with female frailty and male sufferers of the disease were also tainted with accusations of feminised weakness and a lack of manly nerves.

As a result of these theories, mind doctors were concerned with ensuring the regularity of the uterine system, believing that any stoppage, blockage, or over-stimulation could result in terrible consequences. Treatments for female madness were thus often designed to have a direct impact on this part of the body, intended to regulate and control the reproductive functions. These ranged from enforced bed rest (to conserve nervous energy) to the surgical removal of the clitoris or ovaries (Frampton 2018). In addition to cures given to lunatics of both sexes, such as cold-water baths, doctors might apply leeches to the abdomen or give medicine to encourage menstruation. Emotional symptoms were also closely watched, with the exhibition of sexual feelings in female patients regarded as a sign of illness. Mind doctors advised restrictions on behaviour, cautioning against any activity that might upset the delicate balance of reproductive and mental health. More often than not, this required female patients to rest and recuperate through focussing on their feminine duties. Women should avoid over-work, particularly of an intellectual kind, be wary of prolonged physical activity, or strong emotional excitement, and in general remain securely within the serene comforts of the home. As Showalter has argued, 'Victorian psychiatry defined its task with respect to women as the preservation of brain stability in the face of almost overwhelming physical odds. [...The aim was to] help a woman resist the stresses of her body and the weaknesses of her female nature' (Showalter, p. 74).

Such recommendations demonstrate the slippage between cultural attitudes to women and medical theories about the female mind. Although the shifting paradigm of madness made the reproductive hypothesis of female insanity possible, the central importance of these organs to women's mental health and the inferences drawn from this were clearly driven by ideas beyond physiological psychology. Medicine is often thought of as an objective and truth-oriented discipline, yet it is inextricably linked with the cultural and social discourses which influence (either subconsciously or overtly) those who practise in the field (Jordanova 1989). Medical theories about the human body therefore often reflect the dominant belief systems of the society in which they were formed, as well as playing an active part in the making of these beliefs. Indeed, James Secord (2004) has argued that the culture in which scientific work is done is inseparable from the production of knowledge itself. Psychiatry gave scientific validity to existing beliefs about the role of women in society as wives and mothers. The reproductive basis of all theories of female madness only made sense, after all, if reproductive function was of fundamental significance to the female body and mind, logical only when placed in the context of nineteenth-century ideologies of gender that saw women's maternity as their primary purpose.

Scholarship on female madness is supported by studies on the ideology of femininity in the nineteenth century, which emphasise the importance of the reproductive body to women's role in society. Sally Shuttleworth has demonstrated that throughout Western culture 'the male/female divide has operated as a crucial site of ideological deployment' on which the material conditions of society have been shaped (Shuttleworth 1996, p. 84). Shuttleworth argues that during the nineteenth century, this male/female binary became 'strengthened, particularised and codified' around the body, becoming a division based primarily on sex difference (Shuttleworth 1996, p. 84). The reproductive system was foregrounded as a crucial site of meaning for women. As Mary Poovey has shown, this conceptualisation of gender 'underwrote an entire system of institutional practices and conventions at mid-century, ranging from a sexual division of labour to a sexual vision of economic and political rights' (Poovey 1988, p. 8–9). The Victorian concept of women as self-sacrificing, maternal and affectionate was accounted for and reinforced by the supreme importance of their reproductive role as mother.

These beliefs originated in a Christian Evangelical tradition which saw female purity and the maternal role as God-given. With such innate characteristics, there could be no better place for women than in the domestic sphere, raising a family. Ben Griffin has described how Evangelicals believed that the 'development of a [Christian] society that was moral and virtuous' depended on 'a particular set of domestic practices' which ensured that religion was part of everyday life (Griffin 2012, p. 39). From the late-eighteenth century onwards a liberal economy of competition came to dominate the public sphere and virtue began to be located in the domestic world: 'because evangelicals saw the public world of work and politics as a place of temptation, greed and vice, they valued the home as a refuge from these sins and increasingly sought to separate public and private spheres' (Griffin 2012, p. 39–40). Men were 'better able to cope with the trials of the public sphere, while women were supposed to maintain their purity by remaining in the private sphere, where they could create a domestic environment in which family religion could prosper' (Griffin 2012, p. 40). Middle and upper-class women were the guardians of the home. They were seen to embody its virtues, exerting a moral influence on society through their caregiving role as wives and mothers. Dependent on men for subsistence, the labour they contributed to society was therefore emotional and affective. However, middle and upper-class women—and specifically their reproductive bodies—continued to function as part of the capitalist cash nexus through their role as child bearers within marriage, which facilitated the distribution of wealth and property through patrilineal kinship systems.

These ideas took on a novel aspect during the nineteenth century through the association of reproductive difference with the capacity of the body for health. The male body was viewed as strong, healthy and powerful whilst the female body tended to sickness. The sheltered lifestyle of middle-class women was seen as the natural consequence of their weak feminine constitution (Delamont and Duffin 1978). So entrenched were these beliefs that science itself appeared to support the case for women's domestic role. Eagle Russett has shown how studies on evolution, in particular Darwin's *The Descent of Man*, provided a 'starting point for a psychology of sex difference' that theorised man's 'courage, pugnacity, energy' and 'higher intellectual faculties,' in contrast to woman's 'powers of intuition, of rapid perception' and 'of imitation' (Eagle Russett 1989, p. 40–41). The inferior characteristics of women were accounted for by the principle of recapitulation: ontogeny recapitulates phylogeny. Every individual organism 'repeats in its own life history the life history of its race, passing through the lower forms of its ancestors on its way to maturity' (Eagle Russett 1989, p. 50). This theory explained why women were apparently less developed than men, with their weaker body and childish psychology: their growth was arrested at an earlier stage of ontogenetic development. Sexual selection was understood to be the process by which female development had become stunted. Darwin described how the timidity and simple-mindedness of women was a result of their role as reproductive partner. 'Men laboured for subsistence,' whilst women bore children (Eagle Russett 1989, p. 82). Over time, this had encouraged the evolutionary persistence of the select characteristics useful for these roles. The natural sciences therefore served to enforce and affirm a medical view of women as not only tied to their bodily cycles but tethered to the sheer weight of centuries of limited evolutionary development.

However, despite fears about the damage to their health, many women did work. Middle-class women engaged in the complex labour of running a household of servants and children or took to the streets visiting the poor or sick (Rendall 1990; Gleadle 2001). In the second half of the century, women fought for the right to education and gained entry to certain spheres of work, most notably the teaching, nursing and medical professions (Burstyn 1980; Levine 1994; Rowold 1996, 2011). Likewise, working-class women, who through economic necessity did gruelling work for low pay as domestic servants, factory girls and farm labourers, did not fit with the ideology of fragile femininity and their presence was often ignored in discussions of ideal womanhood. As Duffin suggests, 'the contradiction between the myth of woman and the reality' created a 'dual view of women in which their health was not only related to their sex but also linked to class' (Duffin 1979, p. 29–30). Working-class women represented a danger to true, pure womanhood: 'a potential source of sickness to others' (Duffin 1979, p. 30).

Sickening rather than sick, working-class women's freedom of movement outside of the home suggested loose morals. This was often understood as a sexual vulnerability, either to seduction (particularly by men of a higher class) or temptation to prostitution. Women who exhibited sexual desire, particularly in an assertive manner, were thought to be unwell, either morally or mentally. Unruly female sexual desire was the dark side of the influence of the reproductive organs on women's minds. There was thus a paradox inherent in nineteenth-century ideologies of femininity, between maternal innocence and sexualised temptress, which was often articulated through class. These working-class women, whose very existence challenged the ubiquity and thus the essentialism of the angel at the hearth, were rigorously policed through cultural shaming as well as legislative action.

It was this complex web of ideas about women—their maternal nature, physical and intellectual vulnerability and latent sexuality—that provided a conceptual basis for theories of female insanity in the nineteenth century. If evolutionary science provided proof that these gender norms were natural, medicine sought to explain how female physiology supported traditional sex roles. Such arguments foregrounded the reproductive system and rationalised women's role as wife and mother as rooted inevitably in anatomy, reinforcing a social ideology of sex difference. Historians like Showalter have argued that the relationship between nineteenth-century gender norms and psychiatric theories of female insanity is best thought of in this way, as socio-cultural ideas about sex difference influenced medical diagnoses and treatments for mentally ill women.

The Formation of Gendered Psychiatric Theories

However, this book argues that psychiatric theories of the female mind were shaped by *both* the scientific and the social climate in which they were formed. The shift from a spiritual to a physiological paradigm of human psychology, in combination with ideologies of femininity which emphasised women's maternal role, facilitated the creation of a model of the female mind grounded in reproductive biology. The social importance of women's reproductive capacities led to the prominence of the uterus and ovaries in theories of female insanity which looked for an explanation for mental disease in the body. It was thus only through the development of a medical approach to madness that such theories were conceptually viable.

These scientific and cultural influences were brought together through the need of the growing psychiatric profession to establish a theoretical basis for the medical treatment of insanity. Physician superintendents were required to justify their position by demonstrating effective treatment of their patients based on medical expertise, despite their lack of understanding of the aetiology and pathology of insanity during this period. They therefore needed to formulate a concept of mental disease which would function as the epistemological basis of these treatments. Searching for a theory of the female mind which made sense in the absence of pathological evidence, doctors combined what they already knew about the female body with contemporary knowledge about the physiology of the mind. This new clinical model was informed by the up-to-date psychology and physiology of the time, as well as the culture of the individuals practicing in the field. The professionalisation of the discipline was therefore integral to how such theories were formed. Any account of nineteenth-century beliefs about the female mind must consider the growth of psychiatry as a profession alongside cultural attitudes to women.

This book traces the merging of science and culture in the development and deployment of psychiatric theories about women's madness through their primary site of production: the text. Writing was a fundamental part of professional practice in nineteenth and early twentieth-century psychiatry, and crucial to the formation, consolidation and communication of knowledge in an emerging discipline. Scientific and medical writing is not simply a textual representation of a field practised elsewhere but rather an important part of the practice itself, playing a significant role in meaning-making. By revealing the textual conditions in which psychiatric knowledge was produced, it will be possible to make the process through which gendered beliefs about the female mind were formed, tangible and concrete.

The rise of psychiatry as a profession was coincident with a vastly expanded press and reading public. Matthew Rubery has shown how the nineteenth century was an age of transformation, in which a '"reading nation"' was born (Rubery 2009, p. 9). The repeal of the taxes on knowledge, advances in communications and print technologies, and the expansion of education meant that by the end of the century 'virtually everyone read books, magazines, and newspapers to some extent' (Rubery 2009, p. 9). This 'profoundly altered the individual citizen's relation to public life' and the way in which information and knowledge were shared (Rubery 2009, p. 9). Publications became crucial to the disciplinary building activities of the scientific and medical professions. As several scholars have shown (Bynum et al. 1992; Peterson 1992; Mussell 2007; Csiszar 2018; Dawson et al. 2020; Frampton and Wallis 2021; Moulds 2021), by mid-century the publication of texts such as treatises, textbooks, journal articles and society papers was the primary way in which disciplines established their claims to expertise, and practitioners built professional reputation and communities. Writing was also increasingly important to clinical practice, with institutional reports, logbooks and case histories an integral part of patient care and hospital management (Montgomery Hunter 1991; Riha 1995; Porter 1999; Charon 2001; Gills 2006; Hurwitz 2017).

Through examining written discourse, we can therefore understand how theories about the female mind developed during this period. In fact, it is through writing that such theories were created, the text itself being the site of transformation in which medical knowledge, gendered beliefs and the needs of the profession meet. The diverse ways in which psychiatric theories were presented textually altered how such ideas were articulated and understood, as genre and textual form shaped what information was conveyed and to whom. These textual features were determined by the professional context of psychiatric practice, revealing how writing (and therefore theories) about the female mind were impacted by the specific concerns of a discipline in its infancy. The professionalisation of psychiatry influenced the kinds of texts in which these theories were written, the needs of individual authors and the field as a whole directing choices made about genre and place of publication, which in turn shaped the language used to describe women's minds. It is only through placing each text in its full context that a nuanced understanding of nineteenth-century beliefs about the female brain can be achieved.

This book will therefore consider how the development of psychiatry as a discipline, alongside the emergence of a physiological model of the mind, influenced both the content of ideas about female insanity and their articulation in print. It will examine how genre, language, authorship, readership and circumstances of production (such as publishing history) contributed to the formulation and communication of these theories. Genre, for example, was regulated by the desires of the nascent profession for growth and legitimacy, and in turn placed limitations on the information contained within the text. These limitations were imposed through the genre's formal characteristics. Caroline Levine has put forward a useful definition of form as 'all ordering principles,' arguing that form shapes content and meaning within a text (Levin 2005, p. 22). It is the 'peculiar constraints and possibilities that different forms afford,' carried with them 'as they move across time and space,' that dictates what a genre is 'capable of doing' (Levine 2005, p. 25). Levine also contends that the linguistic and literary features of a text are shaped by the social, political and economic forces at work in its context (Levine 2005, p. 29). Form is therefore intrinsically linked to the materiality of the text as printed object. Scientific and medical writing is impacted by the contextual influences common to printed material at large, as well as disciplinary influences, and such circumstances dictate what knowledge is presented and how. This context is often specific to genre; the editorial stance, market audience and cost of publication of a medical journal (covered in Chapter 5) are likely to differ in both kind and importance from a professional textbook (discussed in Chapter 2). There are thus intrinsic social values embedded in genre which are symbolised, deployed and made tangible in the text.

An examination of genre is crucial in reconstructing the role of literature within a society (Bennett 1982; Turner 2000; Mussell 2007; Taavitsainen et al. 2022). Knowledge of a genre's cultural value allows us to trace the impact a text may have at both an authorial and readerly level. Subtle ideological pressures influence the working practices of writers as well as the reception and dissemination of a text (Price 2012). Different periodicals, for example, through the cultivation of specific audiences or the publication of certain types of material, held a different status within Victorian culture and thus evoked particular identities for the reader or writer. The *Fortnightly Review*, which carried mind doctor Henry Maudsley's infamous article on the female mind (covered in Chapter 3), was a periodical marketed at a well-to-do audience with a reputation for intellectual content. This reputation was conferred onto the material published within its pages, giving Maudsley and his article prestige. It is therefore possible to see how written discourses are traceably bound up in the belief systems of the society in which they are made and how texts in turn influence the making of ideas. Even scientific and medical texts must be thought of as products of the culture in which they are written.

Language is also integral to meaning-making within writing, and how the female mind is defined semantically has the power to alter readers' perceptions. The work of Mikhail Bakhtin (1981) is useful in thinking about how the different linguistic properties of texts shape ideas. Bakhtin describes language as a 'social phenomenon' (Bakhtin 1981, p. 259). He argues that it is not only a 'system of linguistic norms' and 'abstract grammatical categories' but a 'world view' which is 'ideologically saturated' (Bakhtin 1981, p. 270–271). Words can therefore shift the conception of their object through use by different writers in different literary forms, for different purposes; laden as they are with cultural and social significance. For example, writing for and by a professional audience often put forward a narrower linguistic representation of female insanity than writing intended for a lay readership. Clinical terminology constrained descriptions of the female brain in a manner which often erased the interior experience of mentally ill women (see Chapter 2). In contrast, writers outside of the medical profession placed psychiatric theories in a social context which is absent from professional texts (Chapter 3). These theories were often adapted and corrupted in non-medical discourse, as the developing profession struggled to maintain jurisdiction over the knowledge it produced. New authors, genres and context made space for new possibilities of meaning, shaped through diverse language.

It is therefore important to see nineteenth-century ideas about the female mind as always in flux, with writing as both a vehicle for their communication and a continuous and active force in their making. Theories of female insanity are a part and product of the texts in which they appear. This book will therefore investigate two forms of written discourse which, together, were integral to the practice of psychiatry during this period: periodicals and clinical literature. Clinical writing such as textbooks and institutional records was the site where theories and methodologies were articulated and recorded. Periodical publications were the primary method of establishing professional identity and communicating findings. Through these two avenues, writing was fundamental to how psychiatric knowledge was retained, developed and shared.

As psychiatry professionalised over the course of the nineteenth century, record keeping became increasingly important to clinical practice, with patient data being charted in case notes. Institutional records were also kept, to monitor patient populations, admissions and recoveries (or deaths). From 1845 English law enforced the keeping of casebooks in county asylums. These served a dual purpose of both aiding government inspection of the new hospitals and encouraging a scientific methodology in the treatment of the insane. This mirrored advancements in medicine at large. Historians such as W. F. Bynum (1994), German E. Berrios and Hugh Freeman (1991, 1996), Roy Porter (1999), and Michel Foucault (2003), have charted the nineteenth-century development of the anatomical-clinical approach to medical practice. Anatomical-clinical medicine raised the epistemological value of observation and investigation in identifying disease, making use of increased knowledge of anatomy and pathology. This was often at the expense of patient's reported experiences, which were of reduced importance in diagnosis. As Porter has shown, the new aim of medical practitioners was to 'identify, record, and analyse symptoms' to 'determine deviations from the norms demonstrated by physiological research' (Porter 1999, p. 561). Under this new paradigm, medical record keeping of all kinds was vital to physicians' ability to gather clinical data and draw conclusions from their findings. They were thus instrumental to the implementation of anatomical-clinical methodologies in the asylum and hospital.

Clinical records were (and are) documents which shape doctors' practice, guiding thinking about patients and disease, as well as revealing the pre-existing beliefs of individuals and the medical profession (Lazenby Craig 1987, 1991). As Guenter B. Risse and John Harley Warner have shown, clinical records are 'surviving artefacts of the interaction between physicians and their patients in which individual personality, cultural assumptions, social status, bureaucratic expediency, and the reality of power relationships are expressed' (Risse and Warner 1992, p. 189). They are texts which convert 'complex clinical perceptions of illness into written narratives,' the form of the record both enforcing a particular selection and therefore interpretation of the data collected (Risse and Warner 1992, pp. 189–190). As Risse and Warner argue, 'reading and interpreting the patient record as a distinct literary text prompts questions of structure and terminology, style and tone, authorship and audience,' from which 'it is possible to retrieve the cultural, institutional, and professional perceptions [and] values' reflected in and encoded by such writing (Risse and Warner 1992, p. 191).

Case notes, for example, were a way of monitoring patient progress, but the way in which they were laid out and formalised, filled in, and consumed was important in shaping knowledge making practices within nineteenth-century hospitals and asylums. They can also reveal a lot about how doctors and attendants thought of their patients. Jonathan Andrews has shown how asylum case notes were shaped by changes in clinical practice throughout the Victorian period, and how they can be a useful source for the uncovering of patient experience as well as 'the preoccupations of the Asylum's medical regime' (Andrews 1998, p. 255). Likewise, admissions registers, as Risse and Warner note, can reveal much about 'contemporary social life and can reflect how local communities [...] defined insanity,' as they often 'recount in great detail the patient's behaviour prior to institutionalisation, including information provided by relatives and friends' (Risse and Warner 1992, p. 186). Some registers were formatted as a pre-designed table which guided the doctors thinking as well as his recording of the facts of patients' admissions. Findings gleaned from analyses of these records were later published in textbooks and treatises. Such texts helped to establish consensus in psychiatry and learnt authority and legitimacy to the medical care of the insane by replicating textual practices used to communicate knowledge in other, well-established, disciplines (Chapter 2).

Psychiatric knowledge was also communicated through periodical publications. As Alex Csiszar has argued, by the end of the century, periodicals (and the scientific paper in particular) became the 'chief avenue by which [practitioners could] make the results of their research into public knowledge claims' (Csiszar 2018, p. 4). These specialist journals also served the purpose of 'demarcat[ing] true practitioners from others,' helping to establish a professional identity for the discipline and its practitioners (Csiszar 2018, p. 8). The first specialist periodicals in psychiatry were founded during this period. The major professional organisation in the field, the Medico-Psychological Association, produced its own *Journal of Mental Science* from 1853, which was managed and edited by prominent members of the Association (Anger 2009). This periodical became an important tool for practitioners to develop their professional reputation, through publishing their clinical findings, and for the discipline itself to form a sense of community, particularly as the journal published the papers and minutes of MPA meetings and kept readers' abreast of news and appointments within the field (Chapter 5).

As Gowan Dawson et al. have argued, scientific and medical periodicals 'played a crucial role in constructing, negotiating, and disrupting [...] communities' of practitioners in the nineteenth century, serving as a visible site of disciplinary identity as well as the practical means of communication between members of the same field (Dawson et al. 2020, p. 5). Alison Moulds has also demonstrated the importance of periodicals in developing a professional identity for individual medical practitioners as well as groups. She argues that practitioners saw the press as the space in which to engage in and define 'questions of medical practice and professionalism,' crucial to the shaping of their sense of self (Moulds 2021, p. 4). Medical men and women were also 'actively involved in textual production and consumption as editors, contributors, correspondents, readers, authors, and reviewers' (Moulds 2021, p. 4). These practices were viewed as an integral part of the professional activities of the medical practitioner. Indeed, 'medical journals self-consciously positioned themselves as important mechanisms for keeping readers informed [...] and developing professional networks' (Moulds 2021, p. 6).

Periodicals were also places where the public could engage with (and get involved in) science and medicine (Cooter and Pumphrey 1994; Cantor et al. 2004; Dawson et al. 2020). Scientific periodicals aimed at non-specialist audiences were common, and as Sally Shuttleworth (2020) and Sally Frampton (2020) have demonstrated, medical practitioners often utilised periodical spaces to communicate with lay audiences. Although nineteenth-century mind doctors did not tend to publish widely in the press (as will be shown in Chapter 3), plenty of public discussion on the discipline (its institutions, diagnoses and treatments) occurred in a wide range of general periodicals. This, as we shall see, allowed the beliefs of mind doctors to be challenged. Both general and specialist periodicals are a key source for understanding how psychiatric theories were raised and responded to both within and outside of the profession.

These two written discourses thus encompass all the major avenues which the psychiatric profession used to think about the mind and are crucial to understanding nineteenth-century theories of female insanity within their intellectual context. This book will take a holistic approach, often examining periodicals and clinical literature side-by-side, and will utilise an interdisciplinary methodology, reading sources as texts whilst placing them within the historical context of psychiatric practice. In doing so, it will analyse how these different forms of writing, each crucial to knowledge-making in the developing discipline, affected the formation of gendered theories of women's minds, variously reinforcing or challenging the reproductive basis for female insanity.

Chapter by Chapter Outline

Before beginning, it is worth pausing to note the terminology which will be used throughout this book, as in the nineteenth century the names used for the mind sciences and those who practised them were fluid. Just as the field changed over the century, so did the various expressions used to categorise physicians who treated the brain. From the pejorative mad doctor to the nouveau alienist, those within and outside of the profession used multiple words to denote who was doing the science, and exactly what kind of science was being done. This book is concerned with the theory and treatment of mental illness in the nineteenth and early twentieth centuries, and the medical doctors who worked within this field. Although there was overlap between the study of insanity, psychology and neurology as a science of the function of the brain, there existed a distinct community of those who cared for the mad. This book therefore uses the term 'psychiatry' to refer to the profession and practice of this kind of medicine, as even though the term was not widely in use until the twentieth century, the subject of this research is the beginnings of what is understood as the discipline today. In reference to the medical men (and women) who thought about, wrote about, and attempted to cure insanity, the terms mind doctor and alienist will be used, alongside asylum-specific terms such as medical assistant. All are appropriate to the period under discussion.

The primary argument made by this book is that attitudes to the female mind within nineteenth-century psychiatry were shaped through textual practices. There is therefore a textual thread which runs throughout the book. However, the book is structured around the various actors involved in the 'psychiatry universe', with each chapter exploring how a different group engaged with theories of the female mind through one or more textual forms or genres. Covering the decades from the passage of the Lunacy Act in 1845 to the eve of the First World War in 1914, this book investigates beliefs about the female mind during a critical period in the history of psychiatry in Britain, when the discipline was becoming established as a medical speciality. Arranging the chapters in this way enables the book to cover the range of medical writing on women's minds during this period, whilst also highlighting the significance of the professional context in the texts under discussion.

The book begins by defining what the psychiatric profession believed about female insanity, demonstrating how mind doctors established a consensus on these theories through written discourse. It then explores how these ideas developed as they were communicated to, and adapted by, others outside of the profession: first discussing the lay public's engagement with psychiatry and, second, the experiences of patients within the asylum system. Finally, the book explores the impact of gendered beliefs on women working in the psychiatric profession, whose very presence challenged the veracity of sexist theories about the female brain. The chapters flow into one another through a laterally expanding scope (as well as, loosely, advancing chronology). The book progressively explores how ideas about the female mind alter, as we move away from the core site of knowledge articulation, which psychiatric professionals saw as the authoritative theory of their discipline: textbooks. This theory, it turns out, becomes much more unstable once we move beyond the pages of textbooks into public debate, patient experiences, and professional realities, and the various textual forms this entailed.

Chapter 2 This chapter investigates how theories of female insanity were formed and communicated by medical professionals (who were then exclusively male), in the fifty years following the passage of the 1845 Lunacy Act. Psychiatry was in its infancy in the nineteenth century and there was no formalised education in the field; most mind doctors transferred to asylum work after a standard medical degree which contained little teaching in mental disease. In the absence of clinical instruction, psychiatric textbooks had a crucial pedagogic role, both for mind doctors and general practitioners. These textbooks were important in creating a consensus of knowledge within the profession and communicating that knowledge to those in training (as well as medical practitioners outside of the asylum community). This chapter discusses how textbooks imparted knowledge of female insanity and shaped treatment practices for women patients, the constraints of the genre influencing what information was presented and how. In particular, the form, narrative structure and semantics of the case history were key to how these texts constructed a theory of female madness which medicalised gender ideology. Designed to replicate the clinical training in psychiatry missing from contemporary medical courses, textbook case histories taught a method of diagnosis and treatment which gave primary importance to reproductive symptoms in female patients. This chapter thus identifies what male mind doctors believed about women's minds, how these theories were communicated to medical professionals, and why this was shaped by the professionalisation of psychiatry as a discipline.

Chapter 3 explores the communication of gendered psychiatric theories outside of the medical profession, examining how the public conceived of and responded to medical beliefs about the female mind. This chapter will examine how periodicals facilitated dialogue, between medical practitioners and lay people, about women's mental capacities. After briefly surveying discussions of female insanity in the popular press, the chapter turns to an unusual example of an article by a mind doctor for a public audience. Henry Maudsley's 'Sex in Mind and in Education', published in the *Fortnightly Review*, applied psychiatric theory to a social question: whether women should be educated in the same way as men. Maudsley's article sparked significant debate in the press. Unlike medical journals, non-specialist periodicals allowed a range of contributors, in particular enabling women to have their views heard. Maudsley thus inadvertently allowed medical knowledge of the female mind to be refuted, expanded and transformed by those outside the profession, the range of textual genres available to writers facilitating a diverse set of responses to his views. The transfer of ideas between professional and lay discourses also highlights the slippage between medical and social beliefs about gender, demonstrating the role ideology had to play in the formation of theories about women's minds.

Chapter 4 returns to the asylum to understand the experiences of female psychiatric patients, investigating whether this reflected the gendered theories set out in textbooks. Taking as a case study Scotland's Crichton Royal Institution in the 1870s and 1880s, the chapter examines how the treatment of women at the asylum was influenced by institutional factors, as well as gendered beliefs. Reading clinical records alongside patients' periodical writing, it explores how the asylum's textual practices both reflected and shaped the institution's approach to insane women. The admissions registers at Crichton Royal demonstrate that the primary factor in decisions made about all patients was the moral management methodology which the institution employed. Nevertheless, the influence of gendered ideologies on this methodology is clear. In the case notes, physicians' gripes were transformed into clinical practices; the institution's moral methodology reinforced gendered standards of good behaviour for female patients, such as quietness and meekness. However, this methodology also meant that patients engaged in therapeutic employments which allowed them a significant amount of agency. One such employment was the asylum's periodical, the *New Moon*, which patients wrote, published and edited. Designed to mould patients' intellect, the periodical was also a much-valued part of asylum life for many and an important space for personal expression. Crucially, women were included in this intellectual endeavour and the periodical gave them a public platform of surprising equality. This suggests that the experiences of female asylum patients were nuanced, varying between and even within individual institutions.

Chapter 5 turns away from discussions of insanity to examine how beliefs about the female mind impacted a different group of women involved with the psychiatric profession: those who worked within the field. As female doctors began to enter psychiatric practice at the turn of the twentieth century, they had to contend with gendered biases like those faced by women patients. Following the life and writing of Dr Helen Boyle, one of the first women to work within an asylum in England, this chapter investigates how her sex impacted her career trajectory. Boyle used textual practices to skilfully manipulate contemporary concepts of femininity and claim a place for herself within the psychiatric profession, taking advantage of the developing nature of her discipline to make advances as a woman. Using a two-pronged approach, Boyle implemented separatist tactics in setting up her own groundbreaking female-led mental health institution (the Lady Chichester Hospital), promoting her vision through the hospital's annual reports. Meanwhile, she employed an inclusionary approach in her periodical publications to garner support from the male establishment through articles in the *Journal of Mental Science*. In the former strategy she utilised stereotypes of her gender but in the latter effaced her sex completely. The written discourses in which she participated gave her the power to shape others' responses to her role as a female mind doctor.

In the *Chapter 6*, this book returns to the historiography of psychiatry. This chapter discusses the early work of the anti-psychiatrists alongside more recent studies (on asylums in particular), which refute the social control model and argue that the treatment of women in psychiatric care during the nineteenth century was not overtly gendered or coercive. Considering these studies, this chapter explores why ideas about the female brain (which this book has shown were clearly gender specific) might have differed from actual clinical practice (a conclusion reinforced in Chapter 4). The conclusion argues that this apparent difference is a skewed perception created by the binary thinking which characterises much of the historiography of psychiatry: such studies often claim that Victorian mind doctors were either wholly bad or good. This provides an opportunity to think critically about the field in which this book is positioned and understand why such binaries have persisted, without returning to them. The emotive relationship we have with nineteenth-century psychiatry, on account of the similarities and continuity between historic and present-day practices, may have influenced historians' judgement.

This book will therefore not only close a gap in our knowledge of Victorian beliefs about the female mind, revealing how these ideas were constituted and contested, but will re-evaluate our perceptions of nineteenth-century psychiatry as a discipline. The clinical methodologies of the discipline were shaped by multiple influences: the culture and society in which they were produced; the expansion of medical knowledge of the human brain and nervous system; and the developing profession's attempts to meet contemporary expectations about legitimate medical practice. Psychiatric theories of female insanity, like all other scientific and medical knowledge, were a product of the holistic context in which they were formed.

References

Published Sources

Andrews, Jonathan. 1998. Documents and Sources: Case Notes, Case Histories, and the Patient's Experience of Insanity at Gartnavel Royal Asylum, Glasgow, in the Nineteenth Century. *Social History of Medicine* 11: 255–281. https://doi.org/10.1093/shm/11.2.255.

Andrews, Jonathan, and Anne Digby, ed. 2004. Sex and Seclusion. In *Class and Custody*, ed. Jonathan Andrews, Anne Digby, Jonathan Andrews, and Anne Digby, 223–248. New York: Rodopi.

Anger, Suzy. 2009. Journal of Mental Science (1853-). In *Dictionary of Nineteenth-Century Journalism in Great Britain and Ireland*, ed. by Laurel Brake and Marysa Demoor, 325. Ghent: Academia Press.

Appignanesi, Lisa. 2009. *Mad, Bad, and Sad: A History of Women and the Mind Doctors from 1800 to the Present*, 2009. London: Virago.

Arieno, Marlene A. 1989. *Victorian Lunatics: A Social Epidemiology of Mental Illness in Mid-Nineteenth-Century England*. London: Associated University Presses.

Bakhtin, Mikhail. 1981. *The Dialogic Imagination: Four Essays*, ed. by Michael Holquist, trans. by Caryl Emerson and Michael Holquist. Austin: University of Texas Press.

Bartlett, Peter, and David Wright. 1999. *Outside the Walls of the Asylum: The History of Care in the Community, 1750–2000*, 1999. London: Athlone Press.

Bennett, Tony. 1982. Media, 'Reality', Signification. In *Culture, Society and the Media*, ed. by Michael Gurevitch et al, 285–306. London: Methuen, 1982.

Berrios, German E., and Hugh Freeman, ed. 1991. *150 Years of British Psychiatry, 1841–1991, Vol. I* London: Gaskell.

Berrios, German E., and Hugh Freeman, eds. 1996. *150 Years of British Psychiatry, 1841–1991, Vol.* II London: Athlone Press.

Bourne Taylor, Jenny. 2010. Body and Mind. In *The Cambridge Companion to English Literature, 1830-1914*, ed. by Joanne Shattock, 184-204. Cambridge: Cambridge University Press.

Brown, Michael. 2006. Rethinking Early Nineteenth-Century Asylum Reform. *Historical Journal* 49: 425–452. https://doi.org/10.1017/S0018246X06005279.

Burstyn, Joan N. 1980. *Victorian Education and the Ideal of Womanhood*. London: Croom Helm.

Bynum, William F. 1994. *Science and the Practice of Medicine in the Nineteenth Century*. Cambridge: Cambridge University Press.

Bynum, William F., Stephen Lock, and Roy Porter, eds. 1992. *Medical Journals and Medical Knowledge: Historical Essays*. Abingdon: Routledge.

Bynum, Wiiliam F., Michael Sheperd, and Roy Porter, ed. 2004. *The Anatomy of Madness: Essays in the History of Psychiatry, Vol. I-III*. London: Routledge.

Cantor, Geoffrey, et al. (eds.). 2004. *Science in the Nineteenth Century Periodical: Reading the Magazine of Nature*. Cambridge: Cambridge University Press.

Charland, Louis C. 2007. Benevolent Theory: Moral Treatment at the York Retreat. *History of Psychiatry*. 18: 61–80. https://doi.org/10.1177/0957154X07070320.

Charon, Rita. 2001. *Narrative Medicine: Honouring the Stories of Illness*. Oxford: Oxford University Press.

Chesler, Phyllis. 2005. *Women and Madness*. Rev. New York: Palgrave Macmillan.

Clark, Michael J. 1981. The Rejection of Psychological Approaches to Mental Disorder in Late Nineteenth-Century British Psychiatry. In *Madhouses, Mad-Doctors, and Madmen: The Social History of Psychiatry in the Victorian Era*, ed. Andrew Scull, 271–312. Philadelphia: University of Pennsylvania Press.

Cooter, Roger, and Stephen Pumphrey. 1994. Separate Spheres and Public Places: Reflections on the History of Science Popularisation and Science in Popular Culture. *History of Science* 32: 237–267. https://doi.org/10.1177/007327539403200301.

Csiszar, Alex. 2018. *Authorship and the Politics of Knowledge in the Nineteenth Century*. Chicago: Chicago University Press.

Dawson, Gowan, Bernard Lightman, Sally Shuttleworth, and Jonathan R. Topham, eds. 2020. *Science Periodicals in Nineteenth-Century Britain: Constructing Scientific Communities*. Chicago: Chicago University Press.

Duffin, Lorna. 1979. The Conspicuous Consumptive: Woman as an Invalid. In *The Nineteenth-Century Woman: Her Cultural and Physical World*, ed. Sara Delamont and Lorna Duffin, 26–56. London: Croom Helm.

Delamont, Sara, and Lorna Duffin, eds. 1979. *The Nineteenth-Century Woman: Her Cultural and Physical World*. London: Croom Helm.

Digby, Anne. 1985. *Madness, Morality and Medicine: A Study of the York Retreat, 1796–1914*. Cambridge: Cambridge University Press.

Digby, Anne. 2004. Moral Treatment at the Retreat, 1796–1846. In *Anatomy of Madness, Vol. II,* ed. By W. F. Bynum, Michael Sheperd, and Roy Porter, 52–72. London: Routledge.

Eagle Russett, Cynthia. 1989. *Sexual Science: The Victorian Construction of Womanhood*. Cambridge: Harvard University Press.

Foucault, Michel. 1999. *Madness and Civilisation: A History of Insanity in the Age of Reason*, trans. by Richard Howard. London: Routledge.

Foucault, Michel. 2003. *The Birth of the Clinic: An Archaeology of Medical Perception,* trans. by A. M. Sheridan. Abingdon: Routledge.

Frampton, Sally. 2018. *Belly-Rippers, Surgical Innovation and the Ovariotomy Controversy.* London: Palgrave Macmillan.

Frampton, Sally. 2020. 'A Boderland in Ethics': Medical Journals, the Public, and the Medical Profession in Nineteenth-Century Britain. In *Science Periodicals in Nineteenth-Century Britain,* ed. Gowan Dawson, et al., 311–336. Chicago: Chicago University Press.

Frampton, Sally, and Jennifer Wallis, eds. 2021. *Reading the Nineteenth-Century Medical Journal.* Abingdon: Routledge.

Gilbert, Sandra M., and Susan Gubar. 1979. *The Madwoman in the Attic: The Woman Writer and the Nineteenth-Century Literary Imagination.* New Haven: Yale University Press.

Gillis, Jonathan. 2006. The History of the Patient History Since 1850. *Bulletin of the History of Medicine.* 80: 490–512. https://doi.org/10.1353/bhm.2006.0097.

Gleadle, Kathryn. 2001. *British Women in the Nineteenth Century.* Basingstoke: Palgrave.

Glover, Mary R. 1984. *The Retreat, York: An Early Experiment in the Treatment of Mental Illness.* York: Ebor Press.

Griffin, Ben. 2012. *The Politics of Gender in Victorian Britain: Masculinity, Political Culture and the Struggle for Women's Rights.* Cambridge: Cambridge University Press.

Hurwitz, Brian. 2017. Narrative Constructs in Modern Clinical Case Reporting. *Studies in History and Philosophy of Science, Part A* 62: 65–73. https://doi.org/10.1016/j.shpsa.2017.03.004.

Jordanova, Ludmilla. 1989. *Sexual Visions: Images of Gender in Science and Medicine Between the Eighteenth and Twentieth Centuries.* Madison: University of Wisconsin Press.

Lazenby Craig, Barbara. 1989. Hospital Records and Record-Keeping, C. 1850-C. 1950, Part I: The Development of Records in Hospitals. *Archivaria,* 29: 57-87.

Lazenby Craig, Barbara. 1991. The Role of Records and of Recordkeeping in the Development of the Modern Hospital in London, England, and Ontario, Canada, c.1890-1940. *Bulletin of the History of Medicine.* 65: 367-397.

Levine, Caroline. 2015. *Forms: Whole, Rhythm, Hierarchy, Network.* Princeton, NJ: Princeton University Press.

Levine, Philippa. 1994. *Victorian Feminism, 1850–1900.* Gainesville: University Press Florida.

Malane, Rachel. 2005. *Sex in Mind: The Gendered Brain in Nineteenth-Century Literature and Mental Sciences.* New York: Peter Lang.

Marland, Hilary. 2004. *Dangerous Motherhood: Insanity and Childbirth in Victorian Britain*. Basingstoke: Palgrave Macmillan.
Marland, Marland. 2012. Under the Shadow of Maternity: Birth, Death and Puerperal Insanity in Victorian Britain. *History of Psychiatry* 23: 78–90. https://doi.org/10.1177/0957154X11428573.
Montgomery Hunter, Kathryn. 1991. *Doctor's Stories: The Narrative Structure of Medical Knowledge*. Princeton: Princeton University Press.
Moulds, Alison. 2021. *Medical Identities and Print Culture, 1830s–1910s*. Cham: Palgrave Macmillan.
Mussell, James. 2007. *Science, Time and Space in the Late Nineteenth-Century Periodical Press: Movable Types*. Aldershot: Ashgate.
Oppenheim, Janet. 1991. *"Shattered Nerves": Doctors, Patients, and Depression in Victorian England*. Oxford: Oxford University Press.
Peterson, Jeanne M. 1994. Medicine. In *Victorian Periodicals and Victorian Society*, ed. by J. Don Vann and Rosemary T. Van Arsdel. 22–44. Aldershot: Scholar Press.
Poovey, Mary. 1988. *Uneven Developments: The Ideological Work of Gender in Mid-Victorian England*. Chicago: Chicago University Press.
Porter, Roy. 1987. *Mind-Forg'd Manacles: A History of Madness in England from the Restoration to the Regency*. Cambridge: Harvard University Press.
Porter, Roy. 1999. *The Greatest Benefit to Mankind: A Medical History of Humanity from Antiquity to the Present*. London: Fontana.
Porter, Roy. 2003. *Madness: A Brief History*. Oxford: Oxford University Press.
Price, Leah. 2012. *How to Do Things with Books in Victorian Britain*. Princeton: Princeton University Press.
Rendall, Jane. 1990. *Women in an Industrialising Society: England, 1750–1880*. Oxford: Basil Blackwell.
Riha, Ortun. 1995. Surgical Case Records as an Historical Source: Limits and Perspectives. *Social History of Medicine* 8: 271–283. https://doi.org/10.1093/shm/8.2.271.
Risse, Guenter B., and Harley Warner. 1992. Reconstructing Clinical Activities: Patient Records in Medical History. *Social History of Medicine* 5: 183–205. https://doi.org/10.1093/shm/5.2.183.
Rowold, Katharina, ed. 1996. *Gender and Science: Late Nineteenth-Century Debates on the Female Mind and Body*. Bristol: Thoemmes Press.
Rowold, Katharina. 2011. *The Educated Woman: Minds, Bodies, and Women's Higher Education in Britain, Germany, and Spain, 1865–1914*. New York: Routledge.
Rubery, Matthew. 2009. *The Novelty of Newspapers: Victorian Fiction After the Invention of the News*. Oxford: Oxford University Press.
Russell, Denise. 1995. *Women, Madness and Medicine*. Cambridge: Polity Press.

Ryland, Rick. 2000. *Victorian Psychology and British Culture, 1850–1880*. Oxford: Oxford University Press.
Scull, Andrew. 1979. *Museums of Madness: The Social Organisation of Insanity in Nineteenth-Century England*. London: Allen Lane.
Scull, Andrew. 1993. *The Most Solitary of Afflictions: Madness and Society in Britain, 1700–1900*. New Haven: Yale University Press.
Secord, James A. 2004. Knowledge in Transit. *Isis* 95: 654–672. https://doi.org/10.1086/430657.
Shepard, Anne. 2004. The Female Patient Experience in Two Late-Nineteenth-Century Surrey Asylums. In *Sex and Seclusion, Class and Custody*, ed. Jonathan Andrews and Anne Digby, 223–248. New York: Rodopi.
Shorter, Edward. 1998. *A History of Psychiatry: From the Era of the Asylum to the Age of Prozac*. Hoboken: Wiley.
Showalter, Elaine. 1987. *The Female Malady: Women, Madness, and English Culture, 1830–1980*. London: Virago.
Shuttleworth, Sally. 1996. *1996*. Charlotte Bronte and Victorian Psychology. Cambridge: Cambridge University Press.
Shuttleworth, Sally. 2020. 'National Health Is National Wealth': Publics, Professions, and the Rise of the Public Health Journal. In *Science Periodicals in Nineteenth-Century Britain*, ed. by Gowan Dawson et al., 337–369. Chicago: Chicago University Press, 2020.
Small, Helen. 1998. *Love's Madness: Medicine, the Novel, and Female Insanity, 1800–1865*. Oxford: Oxford University Press.
Smith, Roger. 1997. *The Fontana History of the Human Sciences*. London: Fontana Press.
Smith, Roger. 2004. The Physiology of the Will: Mind, Body, and Psychology in the Periodical Literature, 1855–1875. In *Science Serialized: Representations of the Sciences in Nineteenth-Century Periodicals*, ed. Geoffrey Cantor and Sally Shuttleworth, 81–110. Cambridge: MIT Press.
Smith-Rosenberg, Caroll, and Charles Rosenberg. 1973. The Female Animal: Medical and Biological Views of Woman and Her Role in Nineteenth-Century America. *Journal of American History*. 60: 332–356. https://doi.org/10.2307/2936779.
Star, Susan Leigh. 1989. *Regions of the Mind: Brain Research and the Quest for Scientific Certainty*. Stanford: Stanford University Press.
Taavitsainen, Irma, et al. (eds.). 2022. *Genre in English Medical Writing, 1500–1820: Sociocultural Contexts of Production and Use*, 2022. Cambridge: Cambridge University Press.
Turner, Mark. 2000. *Trollope and the Magazines: Gendered Issues in Mid-Victorian Britain*. Basingstoke: Palgrave Macmillan.
Ussher, Jane M. 2011. *The Madness of Women: Myth and Experience*. Hove: Routledge.

Wright, David. 2004. Delusions of Gender?: Lay Identification and Clinical Diagnosis of Insanity in Victorian England. In *Sex and Seclusion, Class and Custody*, ed. Jonathan Andrews and Anne Digby, 149–176. New York: Rodopi.

Young, Robert M. 1968. The Functions of the Brain: Gall to Ferrier: 1808–1886. *Isis* 59: 250–268.

CHAPTER 2

The Case of the Madwoman: The Pedagogic Role of Psychiatric Textbooks and the Clinical Presentation of Female Insanity

One of the primary ways in which theories of insanity were established in the Victorian period was through their appearance in psychiatric textbooks. These textbooks began to appear on the market from the late 1840s and were, in essence, manuals of practice. Intended for use by mind doctors, general physicians not trained in the care of the insane, and medical students, they were guides to the diagnosis and treatment of mental disease. Communicating anatomical, pathological, and clinical knowledge, they were designed to fill a gap in the education of medical students and practitioners at a time when the standard certificates did not include training in mental disease. Focusing on psychiatric textbooks published in the fifty-year period following the 1845 Lunacy Act, this chapter offers an analysis of the development of the genre, its readership, and its literary form, in order to understand their pedagogic role within the mind sciences. The lack of clinical training in the discipline meant that textbooks became one of the primary ways in which practitioners and students learnt about insanity during the mid to late nineteenth century. These textbooks were instrumental in the formation of consensus within the discipline, particularly in standardising a foundational concept

M. Chapman, *Writing Women's Madness, 1845–1914*, Palgrave Studies in Literature, Science and Medicine,
https://doi.org/10.1007/978-3-031-97092-4_2

of mental disease that the profession continued to use into the twentieth century.

Textbooks were thus extremely significant for the development of theories of female insanity. As one of the few methods accessible to medical professionals for learning about mental illness, they were influential in establishing theories of the female mind which impacted the treatment of insane women. Psychiatric textbooks medicalised and reinforced gendered social ideologies by connecting mental disturbances in women to reproductive biology. Through their pedagogic role as practical teaching manuals, psychiatric textbooks reproduced cultural ideas about femininity as clinical rules to be put into practice by the reader. These textbooks thus provide further evidence that psychiatric beliefs about the female brain arose from patriarchal assumptions about women's place in society. Crucially, they are also the site where the transformation of such assumptions into medical theories is visible. In particular, one of the defining features of the genre, the clinical case history, was instrumental to this process.

This chapter will first define the boundaries of the textbook genre, along with its aims and audiences, before turning to the content of these books and their representation of female insanity. The form, narrative structure and semantics of the case history were crucial to how these texts constructed a theory of female madness grounded in women's reproductive biology. Significantly, it was through the case history that gendered beliefs about the female mind were turned into elements of clinical practice.

Defining the Genre

Printed texts were an important part of scientific and medical practice in the nineteenth century. Scientific and medical literature made up a substantial proportion of the book industry, at 14% of the output of new titles (Weedon 2003; Csiszar 2018). Several publishing houses dealt exclusively in such books, including the successful publisher, John Churchill. Psychiatric writing was no exception and grew in popularity from mid-century as medical care for the insane was established in legislation and the profession expanded. Mind doctors sought to publish their theories, share their experiences of running an asylum or clinic, and establish reputation in the field. This literature was similar to other medical writing during the period. Works discussing psychiatry commonly appeared as treatises, monographs and published lecture series (from papers originally given at learned societies such as the Royal College of Physicians), all of which were produced in abundance throughout the second half of the nineteenth century. These well-established genres served to circulate knowledge amongst medical practitioners involved in the care of the insane and were important in the establishment of a professional literature for the discipline. The psychiatric textbook developed from the 1840s as a new, specialist genre, though they emulated the form of textbooks published in other fields of medicine.

Between 1845 and 1895 over a dozen textbooks were written and published by medical men whose daily lives involved the care of the insane (Table 2.1). Intended as manuals for the treatment of insanity, they approached the subject from a clinical point of view, describing mental disease from an anatomical, pathological, and diagnostic perspective. John Charles Bucknill and Daniel Hack Tuke, with the publication of their *Manual of Psychological Medicine* in 1858 (Beveridge 1998), claimed to have produced the first psychiatric textbook in response to the 'want for a systematic treatise on insanity, adapted to the use of students and practitioners in medicine' (Bucknill and Tuke 1858, p. iii). The *Manual* was formative for the genre and much more comprehensive than any such work previously published. It was recognised by the psychiatric profession as the go-to text for nearly the next thirty years and became known as the 'classical manual' amongst mind doctors (Bevan Lewis 1889, p. vii). However, earlier works of a similar nature did exist. John Burdett Steward, Joseph Williams, and Daniel Noble had all produced texts in the late 1840s and early 1850s, intended as guides to mental disease for the student and physician. In addition, Robert Brudenell Carter published an extensive treatment manual for hysteria in 1853. These works were published as doctors began to search for more useful formats than the treatise for imparting clinical knowledge.

Over the three decades following the appearance of the *Manual* several textbooks were published that followed a similar formula and a recognisable genre emerged. By the 1870s, mind doctors were writing intentionally within this genre, often stating in the preface to their work that it be understood and read as having 'the character of a text-book' (Fielding Blandford 1871, p. iii). They also frequently referenced each other's works. William Bevan Lewis, in the preface to his *Text-book of Mental Diseases* (1889), asserted that his text contributed to the 'wealth of available literature in this department,' including the 'admirable

Table 2.1 Psychiatric textbooks published in Britain, 1845–1895[1]

Date of publication	*Author*	*Title*	*Publisher and location*
1845	John Burdett Steward	*Practical Notes on Insanity*	London: Churchill
1852	Joseph Williams	*Insanity, its Causes, Prevention and Cure*	London: Churchill
1853	Daniel Noble	*Elements of Psychological Medicine*	London: Churchill
1853	Robert Brudenell Carter	*On the Pathology and Treatment of Hysteria*	London: Churchill
1858	John Charles Bucknill and Daniel Hack Tuke	*A Manual of Psychological Medicine*	London: Churchill
1860	Forbes Benignus Winslow	*On Obscure Diseases of the Brain and Disorders of the Mind*	London: Churchill
1861	John Millar	*Hints on Insanity*	London: Renshaw
1866	William Henry Octavius Sankey	*Lectures on Mental Diseases*	London: Churchill
1871	George Fielding Blandford	*Insanity and its Treatment*	Edinburgh: Oliver and Boyd
1883	Thomas Smith Clouston	*Clinical Lectures on Mental Diseases*	London: Churchill
1884	George Henry Savage	*Insanity and Allied Neuroses*	London: Cassell
1889	William Bevan Lewis	*A Textbook of Mental Diseases*	London: Charles Griffin
1892	Daniel Hack Tuke (ed.)	*A Dictionary of Psychological Medicine*	London: Churchill

lectures of Dr Blandford' and the 'works of Drs Sankey, Clouston, and Savage' (Bevan Lewis 1889, p. vii). Indeed, psychiatric textbooks were increasingly popular; Bucknill and Tuke's *Manual* (1858), Smith Clouston's *Clinical Lectures in Mental Disease* (1883), Forbes Winslow's *On*

[1] Not included in this analysis, due to its dual focus on both physiology and psychiatry, is Theo B. Hyslop's *Mental Physiology: Especially in its Relations to Mental Disorders* (1895). Hyslop worked at Bethlem Asylum from 1888 to 1911, being promoted from Assistant Medical Officer up to Medical Superintendent. His textbook was priced at 18 s. See Mental Physiology. 1897. *Journal of Mental Science*, 43: 150–152.

Obscure Diseases of the Brain (1860), and Bevan Lewis's *Textbook* (1889) all ran into several editions.

These textbooks differed from treatises in both the breadth and nature of their content. Falling into two broad types, the textbook proper and clinical lectures reformatted for publication, they yet have the same literary features. Treatises were generally confined to the discussion of a single, often novel, finding and approached topics from a purely theoretical point of view. Instead, the textbook aimed to cover the range of disorders under the umbrella of insanity and combined theory with practice. They also rarely delivered new theories; textbooks consolidated knowledge and conveyed an established consensus of professional opinion. Above all, they were intended as educational texts. The genre developed in direct response to a lack of formal provision for education in the discipline, seasoned mind doctors taking it upon themselves to pass on the learnings of their profession.

Textbooks and Education

As medical care for the insane became established in England and Scotland, concern arose within the profession regarding the clinical training of physicians seeking to enter practice in asylums. Medical education had progressed significantly during the first half of the nineteenth century. From 1815, it was compulsory by law to pass an examination before being licensed to practise medicine in Britain, either through a university or college, or through the new Licence of the Society of Apothecaries. On the job training was a requirement of the examination, in the form of a five-year apprenticeship and six months' hospital experience. Medical training in Britain was standardised in 1858 with the establishment of the General Medical Council, which regulated the final examinations of the 19 bodies which then awarded licences (Bonner 2000). However, until the late nineteenth century there was no formal academic course on insanity, nor was the subject a compulsory unit of a medical degree. Education in psychiatry lagged behind that of general medicine, with many practitioners falling into the field and simply learning on the job (Beveridge 1991). Asylum doctors were not required to have specialist training and clinical teaching in psychiatry was fragmentary at best.

In 1827, Alexander Morrison delivered the first lectures on insanity in an unofficial course, as the University of Edinburgh would not allow him to teach at the medical school.[2] From the 1830s to the 1860s, lecturing in psychiatry was generally at the initiative of individual mind doctors, either from their home asylums—such as John Connolly's 1842 lectures at Hanwell—or when they could get medical schools to agree to host the course. From the 1850s, the number of courses available increased, among them W. A. F. Browne's course at Crichton Royal and David Skae's lectures at the Royal Edinburgh Asylum (Crichton Browne 1861). Over the next decade further lecture series were given at London teaching hospitals, such as George Fielding Blandford's course at St. George's, as well as at asylums, such as those given by Thomas Smith Clouston and George Henry Savage (these were afterward adapted for publication as lecture-style textbooks). However, it was not until the 1870s that medical schools began appointing lecturers in mental pathology on a permanent or semi-permanent basis; George Henry Savage's chair in Mental Physiology at Guy's Hospital being the first of its kind in 1871 (Beveridge 1991). The Medico-Psychological Association (a membership organisation for practitioners in the care of the insane) began campaigning for certification in the field and succeeded in inaugurating a Certificate of Efficiency in Psychological Medicine in 1885. Unfortunately, as William Bynum (1991) has demonstrated, the Certificate was not very successful as the examination was too general and was not registrable. It was only in 1893 that the General Medical Council made psychiatric instruction compulsory for all medical students.

Despite the lack of interest from the medical establishment at large, there was a call for better training from within the community of those who cared for the insane. In his youth, as president of the Extraordinary (student) section of the Royal Medical Society of Edinburgh, James Crichton Browne advocated for the inclusion of teaching on mental disease as standard for the British medical degree.[3] In his 1861 speech, published as *The Clinical Teaching of Psychology: A Valedictory Address*, he proposed a course of lectures including class visits to a hospital for the insane. He argued that a growing 'class of medical men having the charge of county, district, or chartered asylums' were entering upon such service without any special preparation for it, a state of affairs that could hardly

[2] These were popular and became an annual commemorative series from 1864: the Morrisonian Lectures, held at the Royal College of Physicians, Edinburgh.

[3] James Crichton Browne later went on to set up an unofficial school of psychiatry at the West Riding Asylum in Wakefield.

be allowed to continue (Crichton Browne 1861, p. 14). In addition, Crichton Browne felt that clinical education in mental disease was imperative for the medical profession as a whole. After the introduction of lunacy certification in 1845, English law required that for an insane person to be admitted to an asylum, two physicians not associated with the institution needed to give their signature of approval (Wright 1998). This resulted in medical men wholly inexperienced in lunacy having a great responsibility for the welfare of insane patients. Crichton Browne stressed that the 'general practitioner in extensive practice must frequently be called upon to decide as to the mental condition of many of his patients,' thus having total control over the 'personal liberty of the individual' (Crichton Browne 1861, p. 13). Clinical instruction in mental disease would provide the practitioner with 'practical knowledge, which enables him to recognise the symptoms of disease,' and furnish him 'with the means of arriving at a sound and just conclusion' (Crichton Browne 1861, p. 13).

Established professionals were also calling for improvements in psychiatric education. Polina Merkulova, in her unpublished MA dissertation *The Making of a Manual* (University of Leeds 2016), has explored how Bucknill and Tuke's textbook arose out of Tuke's experiences of the limited availability of teaching on insanity. In the mid-1850s he taught a short summer course on mental disease at the York Medical School. Merkulova describes his notes for these lectures, pointing out his complaints about the 'misleading assumption that no special learning or expertise is needed' in the practice of psychological medicine (Merkulova 2016, p. 26). Tuke believed that as the fundamentals of the discipline were mostly unknown outside of the professional alienist community, psychiatry seemed to others to be a dubious science. As things stood, the reputation of the budding profession was at risk. He proposed that 'the basic elements of psychiatry should be identified and taught to all medical students, and even be available to the general public in a suitable form' (Merkulova 2016, p. 5). As Merkulova argues, in the absence of formalised academic teaching, writing a textbook was the logical answer to this dilemma: a didactic work would consolidate clinical knowledge in one easily accessible place (Merkulova 2016).

There was thus general agreement amongst the mind doctoring community that training in the care of the insane was needed to secure a better future for the discipline, as well as to ensure that physicians could meet their new legal responsibilities. In the want of any official move to include such training in medical school prospectuses, psychiatric textbooks attempted to fill the gap in the educational market. Many authors prefaced their work by positioning the textbook as the solution to these problems.

In his *Insanity and its Treatment*, Blandford noted the 'few works' which 'exist in our language' suitable for use as class books (Fielding Blandford 1871, p. iii). His aim, in creating 'a handy book concerning insanity [and] written for students,' was to provide a didactic text that copied the form of his lectures at St. George's Hospital (Fielding Blandford 1871, p. iii). Likewise, just over a decade later in 1883, Smith Clouston published his lectures 'as a text-book for my students in the University of Edinburgh,' presenting an 'entirely clinical and practical point of view as desired' by those undertaking the study of medicine (Smith Clouston 1883, p. v). He also stressed the usefulness of his manual for 'busy practitioners,' and his hope that the textbook would 'assist some of my brethren in their treatment of a very obscure and troublesome class of diseases' (Smith Clouston 1883, p. v-vi). Like Crichton Browne, Daniel Noble worried about 'the duty of the ordinary medical attendant of families' to recognise insanity in its 'incipient stage,' and to adopt 'decisive measures' (Noble 1853, p. vi). Such men were unlikely to have any real clinical knowledge of mental disease at all, an 'anomaly [which] becomes still more striking, when the subject is considered from a legal point of view. The personal freedom of individuals can always be taken away, if two medical men certify to the fact of insanity' (Noble 1853, p. vii).

Psychiatric textbooks can therefore be understood as a collective effort to provide educational materials of a clinical nature, a grass-roots response to the dearth of appropriate training in the care of the insane in the mid-Victorian period. This was recognised as a problem for the medical community at large, as the medical care of the insane expanded and it became more necessary—and more likely—for doctors to treat mental disease. Three groups were seen as especially needful for training: medical students just starting on their careers; mind doctors who required access to a consensus of professional opinion; and general physicians, frequently called upon in their daily working lives to diagnose cases of insanity. The textbooks were designed to appeal, and be of use, to all these professionals.

Textbooks and the Medical Community

For textbooks to improve professional knowledge of insanity and its treatment, they had to be read and shared amongst mind doctors and other medical practitioners. By investigating the publication and potential readership of psychiatric textbooks, it is possible to judge the success of these works as pedagogical texts and therefore ascertain how important they were for the nineteenth-century mind sciences. The evidence suggests that these textbooks were widely read and were indeed useful texts for mind doctors, general practitioners, and students alike.

Over two-thirds of the textbooks identified in this chapter were published by John Churchill (later, under the partnership of his sons, J&A Churchill), one of the most prominent medical publishing houses in the nineteenth century. As James Secord has shown, Churchill's shop was 'an informal centre for London medical men' (Secord 2003, p. 113). Churchill was 'intimate with the leading medical authors,' and willing to be 'associated with a variety of "advanced" medical views' (Secord 2003, p. 114). The company produced a huge range of treatises, educational works, popular titles, and journals, but was known for having a curated list including some of the hottest titles on the market. Psychiatric textbooks were only a small part of Churchill's repertoire of publications but their presence on the company's list would have lent the works good repute within the medical community. A Churchill publication was a reliable one and it is possible that textbook authors sought to publish under the house to lend legitimacy and prestige to their work, particularly as they were writing within an emerging discipline.

Psychiatric textbooks were accessible. Churchill and other publishers produced the books in a format and price bracket comparable with other types of medical literature. Bound economically in cloth (the cheapest material for binding), printed on paper that was serviceable rather than luxurious, and arranged in octavo format, the textbooks were reasonably inexpensive. Although certainly not affordable for the lower classes, they were priced at a level to which the middle-class physician could stretch. Unlike the costly three volume novels of the period, which were typically sold at 31s, psychiatric textbooks were marketed as one volume in a medium price bracket. Churchill's psychiatric textbooks cost between 4 and 16s in the 1860s (Fig. 2.1). This indicates that publishers intended them to be purchased by those on a professional salary. As Simon Eliot (2000, 2009) has argued, an increase in real household income between the 1860s and 1890s made titles published between 3s 6d and 10s attainable for most of the middle classes. Although the cost of textbooks sometimes rose above this, they were rarely priced at above 20 per cent of a doctor's weekly income, which tallied to earnings between £2 and £5 over the mid to late nineteenth century. Perhaps something of a considered purchase, they were nevertheless within reach (Altick 1999; St. Clair 2004).

This price bracket was comparable with other types of medical text published during the period: a sample comparison of physiological textbooks published by Churchill between the 1850s and 1860s reveals a similar price point for these works, at around 8s 6d to 12s, rising to 18s at the costliest volume. Textbooks were not new to nineteenth-century medicine and had been a major part of medical writing since at least the early 1800s, which suggests that publishers were matching their pricing of these books with an existing market. The average price of psychiatric textbooks did increase over the course of the period, but this related to the expansion of the text across editions rather than rising costs. Authors often produced larger, more detailed editions after the success of the first (Fig. 2.1). Bucknill and Tuke's 1873 edition of the *Manual* is a good

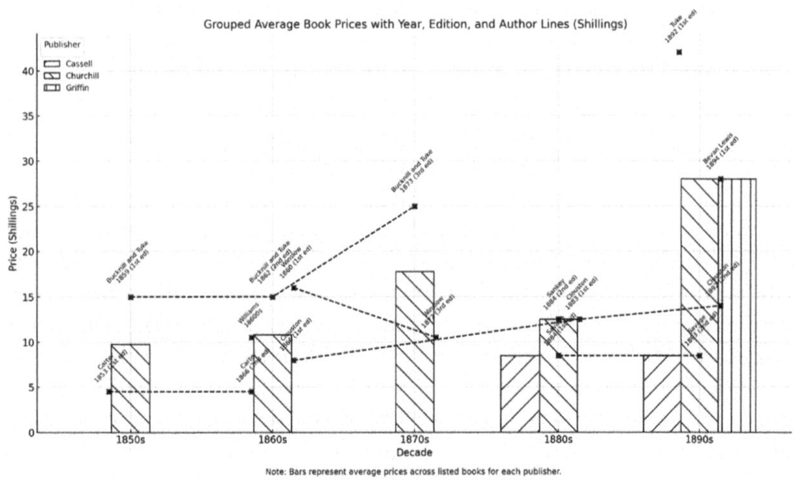

Fig. 2.1 Cost of psychiatric textbooks published in Britain across multiple editions, 1845–1895

example of this, to which illustrations were added. Certain texts were significantly more expensive, such as Tuke's *Dictionary* (which was a large double volume work and not strictly a textbook). However, most were much, much cheaper than the *Dictionary*'s 42s. Affordable editions were also published, with a student market specifically in mind. The publisher Cassell and Company included Savage's textbook within their 'Clinical Manuals for Practitioners and Students of Medicine' series. Bound at a size convenient for the pocket, these sold at 8s 6d each in the 1880s.

In addition, psychiatric textbooks were available to be read in specialist libraries. Students would have been able to access copies held in their school's collection. Medical libraries often held quite a range of textbooks and effort was generally made to keep the collection up to date with new editions. The Royal College of Physicians Library contained a wide selection. The catalogue records for 1912 show that throughout the second half of the nineteenth century, the library acquired nearly every one of the textbooks listed in Table 2.1, barring Smith Clouston's *Clinical Lectures* (Royal College of Physicians of London 1912). The Yorkshire College Medical Department Library (shared with the Leeds and West Riding Medico-Chirurgical Society) (Catalogue of the Joint Library of the Medical Department of the Yorkshire College 1892) and the University College London Medical Library (Catalogue of Books in the Medical and Biological Libraries at University College London 1887) both contain catalogue records for several psychiatric textbooks in up-to-date editions, including works by Blandford, Clouston, Bevan Lewis, Bucknill and Tuke, Noble, and Savage. The presence of manuals of psychiatry in these and similar libraries shows that they were thought necessary additions to collections catering for the medical community. These libraries were not exclusively for mind doctors and the books were thus accessible to those who did not necessarily have direct experience of treating insanity, including students and general practitioners. This indicates that the texts were readily accessible to their intended audience for their intended purpose.

The distribution figures available for the textbooks support this. Churchill's titles were printed in medium-sized runs, with most at between 500 and 750 copies per run (Table 2.2). Alexis Weedon (2003) has shown that, from the mid-nineteenth century onwards, publishers typically printed in runs of around 500–1000 copies to minimise capital tied up in unsold stock. Companies printed short runs of books to avoid heavy outlay and to test the market, preferring to reprint if titles were found to be sufficiently popular. Right from the beginning, psychiatric textbooks were produced in numbers consistent with moderate demand, suggesting that Churchill expected the books to have a ready audience of readers. This is compatible with the demand which mind doctors themselves expressed for such works. Two textbooks were printed at even larger runs in their later editions: Bucknill and Tuke's *Manual* and Clouston's *Clinical Lectures*, at runs of 1000 and 2000 respectively. Significantly, these volumes were printed in editions only a few years apart, indicating that the books were selling out swiftly. As we have seen, the *Manual* was something of a seminal work during the mid-Victorian period, which accounts for its greater popularity. It therefore likely that Clouston's work was also read widely, perhaps even appealing to members of the general public. A run of 1000 in 1896, followed by one of 2000 in 1898, certainly suggests this.

Polina Merkulova, looking at the distribution of Bucknill and Tuke's *Manual*, has pointed out that even a print run of 750 copies was remarkably large considering that 'the membership of the AMOAHI [Association of Medical Officers of Asylums and Hospitals for the Insane, later the Medico-Psychological Association] at the time was only about one hundred and fifty people' (Merkulova 2016, p. 36). She therefore argues that 'the *Manual* reached far beyond the specialist community to other medical practitioners, students and the general public' (Merkulova

Table 2.2 Print runs of Churchill titles across multiple editions, 1845–1895

		1st Edition	*2nd Edition*	*3rd Edition*	*4th Edition*	*5th Edition*
Bucknill and Tuke	**Run**	600	250	750	1000	
	Date	*1858*	*1862*	*1873*	*1879*	
Carter	**Run**	200				
	Date	*1853*				
Clouston	**Run**	750	750	750	1000	2000
	Date	*1883*	*1887*	*1892*	*1896*	*1898*
Sankey	**Run**	500				
	Date	*1866*				
Steward	**Run**	750				
	Date	*1845*				
Winslow	**Run**	750	750			
	Date	*1860*	*1868*			

2016, p. 36). With such sizable print runs it is certainly likely that educated members of the public also read the textbooks, particularly as insanity and its treatment was a hot topic during this period. Records show that the most popular texts were available in non-specialist libraries. The Leeds Central Library, a public lending library which opened in 1884, contains catalogue records for 2 textbooks: Savage's *Insanity* and Winslow's *On Obscure Diseases* (Catalogue of the Central Lending Library 1894). The catalogue for the London Library, which was open to the public but had an upper-class membership, also has records for those textbooks which had the largest distribution figures. Between 1841 and 1909, the library acquired the works of Bucknill and Tuke, Clouston, and Winslow (Hagberg Wright 1909). The presence of these books in non-specialist libraries indicates that there may have been some interest in insanity amongst the non-medical public, but copies of the most famous volumes would have at least been useful as reference books for provincial doctors who may not have had access to medical libraries.

Periodicals from the period also indicate that audiences beyond the medical community would have been aware of the textbooks. As a marketing strategy, publishers like Churchill sent copies of new works to editors for review, in the hopes that they would write favourably about them in their journal. These reviews can tell us something of the response to psychiatric textbooks. A sample search for four popular textbooks, by Bucknill and Tuke, Savage, Winslow, and Bevan Lewis, showed that these titles were reviewed in a range of publications, both medical and non-specialist. The reviews most often appeared under the 'Science News' or 'New Books' section of the periodicals. Reviewers praised the texts for their clear style and insight, and highlighted sections that would be of interest to both the practitioner and public.

For example, the *Athenaeum* praised Bucknill and Tuke's *Manual* as a much looked-for text on insanity. An 1859 review wrote that 'the general public will find Dr Tuke's part written in an agreeable style and devoted to subjects in which all persons living in a civilised country have a greater or lesser interest,' whilst 'the practitioner engaged in the treatment of diseased minds cannot fail to be instructed by the earnest, truthful, and manly spirit in which Dr Bucknill treats his part of the subject' (Medical Books: A Manual of Psychological Medicine 1859). Likewise, the *Edinburgh Review*, discussing Winslow's *On Obscure Diseases of the Brain and Disorders of the Mind* in October 1860, remarked that 'the various forms of cerebral mischief detailed in Dr Winslow's volume' are 'to the general reader as interesting as a romance' (On Obscure Diseases of the Brain 1860, p. 545). To the professional, however, the book is a 'storehouse of fact' (On Obscure Diseases of the Brain 1860, p. 545). In presenting scientific ideas clearly, the textbooks allowed educated, interested people to acquire some knowledge of the field.

Nineteenth-century publishers also advertised heavily in periodicals, devoting a hefty part of the budget for a new book to frequent adverts placed in a range of titles, usually over the first year or two after an edition was published. However, Churchill spent a mammoth £102 6s 6d on Winslow's *Obscure Diseases* in just twelve months (Authors' Ledgers 1845–1900). The publishing house placed adverts for its psychiatric textbooks in numerous publications, ranging from non-specialist periodicals such as the *Literary Gazette*, *Blackwood's Magazine*, *Fortnightly Review*, and *Saturday Review*, to newspapers such as the *Times* and *Telegraph*. Adverts were also frequently placed in medical journals like the *Lancet*, *Medical Times*, *British Medical Journal*, and *Hospital Gazette* (Authors' Ledgers 1845–1900). Churchill followed a standard marketing strategy for the time, hitting all the major periodicals with readerships in the right social bracket, but the financial investment made in these books clearly indicates that the house thought them a valuable part of their list. Members of the medical profession would have certainly come across advertisements placed in the periodicals they read for work or leisure.

Psychiatric textbooks were clearly an important and popular genre of medical literature during this period. If we consider the evident popularity of the textbooks in the context of their educational purpose, it appears that they were proving a valuable and successful alternative to academic teaching in insanity, reaching their intended readerships. In the absence of formalised education in the mind sciences, these works were to prove indispensable in providing the medical community with information about the nature and treatment of mental disease. The popularity of psychiatric textbooks demonstrates that they became foundational texts within the nineteenth-century mind sciences, providing a reliable resource on which clinical practitioners could draw. Their wide acceptance is significant as this shows that the theories the textbooks contained became an established consensus and that the books set a standard for the treatment of insanity.

Textbooks and Clinical Practice

Psychiatric textbooks were especially useful as practical guides to clinical work in the care of the insane, crucially missing from the medical curriculum. Joseph Williams wrote in *Insanity, its Causes, Prevention, and Cure* (1852) of the 'hiatus which has long been known to exist' in the clinical instruction on mental disease: the want of academic teaching in psychiatry had caused a scarcity of this vital aspect of training (Williams 1852, p. x). This was damaging both in regard to practitioners' ability to do their job well and to the reputation of the developing discipline. Textbooks enabled mind doctors to formalise their knowledge, translating on-the-job experience into a coherent narrative which could easily be communicated to readers. Although the textbooks assumed a foundational understanding of anatomy and physiology, mental diseases were explained in a manner that was easy to follow and translate into practice for someone who had little experience treating patients with insanity.

Over the nineteenth century, there was a growing emphasis on an anatomical-pathological approach within medicine, in which psychiatry trailed behind. Roy Porter (1999) has shown that whereas clinical observation had previously been restricted to what could be viewed externally, with advancements in medical technologies symptoms could now be correlated with signs found in the body post-mortem. Knowledge of how internal organs functioned in health (anatomy) and disease (pathology) was key to the understanding of disease. This knowledge was acquired primarily within hospitals, through time spent on the wards. In mainstream medicine, training was 'a matter of drilling students to interpret the signs, sounds, and smells of disease' (Porter 1999, p. 312). In short, tutoring them in clinical judgement. It was on this basis that practitioners could 'develop valuable therapeutic interventions' (Porter 1999, p. 561). Students hoping to study mental disease lacked the opportunity to visit patients as teaching hospitals attached to medical schools did not have psychiatric wards at this time. Williams complained that 'a great deal of practical experience in the management of the patient' is only acquired 'after the medical man has completed his education' and is at work in the asylum (Williams 1852, p. x). This meant that mind doctors began their careers without valuable information on 'important symptoms,' or the knowledge of 'some particular remedy' (Williams 1852, p. x). The inaccessibility of asylums 'for the purposes of clinical study' made any proper attempt at such training even more difficult (Williams 1852, p. x).

There was therefore a strong emphasis on providing this missing practical knowledge within psychiatric textbooks. These textbooks came to be relied upon as clinical manuals which artificially recreated the *in-praxis* experience medical schools would otherwise provide.

Psychiatric textbooks were authored by working professionals, who were best placed to provide the clinical and practical understanding of mental disease which was felt to be missing from medical education. It is this hands-on expertise which, over and above theoretical approaches, is given epistemological value in the textbooks. George Savage wrote in his *Insanity and Allied Neuroses* that he owed it to his 'position as physician to a large hospital to give the younger members of my profession the results of my more than twelve years' experience in Bethlem' (Savage 1884, p. vi). Likewise, Smith Clouston stressed that a textbook must have a 'foundation in the clinical experience of its author,' and appeal 'directly and on all occasions to the facts of disease as seen in actual cases' (Smith Clouston 1883, p. v). Such experiential knowledge was crucial as the textbooks had to function as replacements for time spent on the wards, becoming the primary site of learning for doctors.

Authors of psychiatric textbooks utilised a format familiar to them from textbooks in other disciplines, used during their time in medical school (and in their professional life as medical men). Written in a clear and conversational tone, the textbooks are arranged in easily digestible parts: chapters or lectures, depending on the format, and bitesize subsections. In the lecture-style textbooks, which were adapted from real-life classes given to students, the material has transitioned from oral to written (published) form. The original tone of the lecture is thus partially retained through first-person narration and direct address. Material is also divided into chapters corresponding to individual talks in the series, so that the reader moves progressively towards knowledge through the text in much the same way as in attending a course. Whilst the reference-style textbooks do not divide the material in this way, they do have a rhetorical flair, with the author's voice often coming through the clinical narrative to offer comment or advice. Often, chapters are divided into nosological groups, with each disease or sub-set of diseases falling under separate headings. This increased ease of reference, particularly for those who might wish to confirm their own diagnosis, or who were unsure of how to proceed with treatment. The textbooks are formatted to facilitate the efficiency of reading, with sub-headings and keywords in bold or italic and comprehensive indexes. They also include pedagogic tools, such as statistics, charts and illustrations, to further illuminate complex topics.

In both styles, each chapter guides the reader through discrete sections from anatomy to pathology, diagnosis, and finally treatment. In doing so, the textbooks teach the basics required for a medical understanding of mental disease and focus on the practical issues necessary for dealing with real patients. By moving through these sections methodically, they also follow the progress of a medical course. First, teaching the theory of each disease, the presentation of healthy anatomy and pathological changes occurring under the presence of disease. Next, addressing the practical aspects of medical education, dealing with patients, and how to diagnose and treat the disorder: the disease is described as it would be assessed by a doctor, replicating the stages of patient care textually. The textbooks also contain useful information on day-to-day practicalities, such as pharmacological measurements for drugs used in sedation and guidelines on how to complete a certification of lunacy. One of the key features of these textbooks, which will be discussed in detail below, is the use of clinical case histories to illustrate theories of disease. These cases directly translated clinical experience into print and replaced first-hand knowledge of treating patients on asylum wards. Providing blueprints for the diagnosis of a variety of types of mental illness, they demonstrated common signs of insanity to prepare the reader for similar instances in their own practice. As such, these case histories were key to the formation of students and physicians' understanding of mental disease.

As the primary source of information on insanity both within the mind sciences and the medical community at large, psychiatric textbooks developed a special authority as scientific works. They consolidated existing knowledge of mental disease and the theories they contained became the dominant paradigm of insanity from the mid-nineteenth century onwards. As pedagogic texts, they passed on this paradigm to new generations of doctors. Psychiatric textbooks are therefore a key source for understanding nineteenth-century ideas about the female mind as, amongst other diseases, they highlight what the profession thought important to impart to students and newcomers alike. As this chapter will discuss, the form of the textbooks—directed by their purpose of clinical instruction—shaped the way this knowledge was presented and communicated. Psychiatric textbooks thus also played an active part in the development of these gendered theories.

Female Madness in Psychiatric Textbooks

Historians such as Elaine Showalter (1987), Hilary Marland (2004), and Rachel Malane (2005) have demonstrated that nineteenth-century theories of female insanity linked the reproductive organs, the nerves, and the brain in a sympathetic loop. Mind doctors believed that the reproductive system exerted a tax of energy upon the female constitution which made women especially liable to mental disease, particularly during the periodic crises of reproductive activity. These scholars have argued that such ideas were based in long-standing gendered social ideologies which positioned women's maternal and domestic role at the heart of their identity. They have shown how psychiatry encouraged these ideologies by providing them with a scientific basis and cautioning women against anything which could make them more vulnerable to mental disturbance, such as intellectual work.

However, absent from such studies is an examination of how psychiatric theories of the female mind were formulated and communicated. It is particularly important to discover how gendered social beliefs were combined with medical knowledge in the creation of such theories. The importance of psychiatric textbooks in the knowledge-making processes of the Victorian mind sciences was a major factor in the establishment of a specifically gendered concept of women's madness. Textbooks are a key site where we see this formation in action. Of course, that these were foundational texts for the discipline meant that the ideas they presented were read widely, largely accepted, and translated into practice. However, textbooks were also the space in which doctors articulated and defined the fundamental theories on which their profession was based. We can therefore see *what* mind doctors thought about the female brain and *how* they developed these beliefs.

The representation of women in these textbooks clearly establishes a relationship between social ideologies and theories of the female mind. The reproductive organs are linked to female insanity in all textbooks from this period, though later works present more of a nuanced aetiology as knowledge of the origins of mental disease became more sophisticated; insanity was increasingly seen as the result of several coalescent factors, ranging from moral shocks to organic disease, to heredity. The pathology of disorders also became clinically important from the 1880s onward as doctors became interested in discovering the physiological origin of insanity in the nerves and brain. Like men, women were at risk of all these factors but, as the textbooks demonstrate, they were believed to have an overall greater nervous susceptibility because of their reproductive biology. As George Fielding Blandford commented, 'the sympathetic connexion existing between the brain and the uterus is plainly seen by the most casual observer' (Fielding Blandford 1871, p. 54). The dramatic life cycle changes of menstruation, pregnancy, childbirth and so on, placed female mental stability under special risks: female biology meant that certain periods of a woman's life were 'fraught with greater peril' (Fielding Blandford 1871, p. 56). Psychiatric textbooks set out specific classes of mental disease related to women's reproductive life, such as puerperal mania and climacteric insanity (insanity of menopause). In contrast, there was no concept of male insanity equivalent to that applied to female cases, though certain types of mental disease were recognised as predominantly affecting male patients, such as general paralysis of the insane and spermatorrhoea—a sexual disorder characterised by excessive and involuntary ejaculation.

Doctors generally agreed that women had a lesser capacity to deal with shocks or negative experiences due to their weaker nervous system, though this was not straightforward. The relationship between female reproduction and mental disease is presented within the textbooks as sympathetic (rather than directly causal), and disturbance could be a symptom of insanity or simply an effect of ill-health. Thomas Smith Clouston argued in his *Clinical Lectures on Mental Diseases* that although 'the regular normal performance of the reproductive functions is of the highest importance to the mental soundness of the female, [...] it does not follow from this [that disturbance] caused the insanity in all such cases' (Smith Clouston 1883, p. 510). He complained that 'the constant difficulty the physician has' is to know whether the uterine problem is 'a cause or symptom' (Smith Clouston 1883, p. 510). Attention was also paid to the influence of other factors in exciting lunacy in women, such as domestic strain and the physical exhaustion resulting from repeated child-bearing or prolonged lactation. Regardless, female mental health was seen as precarious: women's biology meant that certain periods of life were 'fraught with greater peril' (Fielding Blandford 1871, p. 56). Significantly, there is little difference, when looking chronologically, between theories of female insanity written either at the beginning or end of our fifty-year period. A specific understanding of female madness, rooted in beliefs about the primacy of women's role as child bearers, remained consistent throughout the century.

Such consistency suggests that these core beliefs were powerful and resistant to change, arguably because of their basis in cultural perceptions of women. However, psychiatric textbooks, in giving scientific validity to misogynistic social ideologies at a time when the epistemological authority of the discipline was on the rise, played a key role in reinforcing their value. The lack of alternative education on insanity and the pedagogic usage of the textbooks encouraged the endurance of these ideas within the profession. The separation of female disorders into their own discrete categories with gender-specific symptoms was a major influence on how doctors thought about women's minds, as it necessitated differentiation between the sexes.

Gendered theories were also incorporated into the most valued component of the textbooks: their clinical instruction. This ensured the permanency of such theories and directly influenced how mind doctors thought about women with mental illness. In particular, a gendered concept of the female mind was propagated through case histories which integrated women's reproductive biology and cultural beliefs about their social role into the clinical pathway. Case histories formalised these gendered ideas and made them crucial to the diagnosis and treatment of any woman presenting as mentally ill. The didactic role of the case history within the textbook was a powerful factor in encouraging the continuity of these theories and ensuring their longevity within the mind sciences and medical community at large.

Clinical Case Histories and the Teaching of Female Madness

By the mid-nineteenth century, clinical case histories were well established as a method of recording medical findings. As Roy Porter (1999) has shown, the case history developed directly in relation to anatomical-clinical medicine. Porter defines this type of medical practice as methods of investigation which 'aim to identify, record and analyse symptoms presented in sickness; determine deviations from the norms demonstrated by physiological research; and on those bases develop valuable therapeutic interventions' (Porter 1999, p. 561). This new approach was characterised by a shift from patient experience to the observations of the physician, as well as an increased specialisation in internal anatomy and pathology. Designed to effectively record and make sense of this kind of information, the case history was the perfect tool for understanding disease within the new paradigm; as Foucault has argued, the case structured medical knowledge through the clinician's gaze (Foucault 2003).

The keeping of case histories became standard on hospital wards from the early 1800s and common practice in psychiatry when the Lunacy Act of 1845 enforced the use of casebooks in county asylums in England (Andrews 1998). The Act marked the transition of insanity from a religious to a medical concern and was the result of a series of legislative moves towards increasing professionalisation within the mind sciences. Casebooks were seen as important as they both facilitated better inspections by the Lunacy Commissioners and symbolised a scientific attitude to mental disease, aligned with the anatomical-clinical model (Andrews 1998). From this time, case histories were an important method of structuring and communicating clinical knowledge. It therefore makes sense that cases were used extensively in nineteenth-century psychiatric textbooks: they were often drawn from the author's own patient records at their home asylum.

Case histories were one of the most valuable educational tools at mind doctors' disposal, as they were an excellent way to recreate clinical experience. Case histories conveyed both theoretical and practical knowledge, reproducing a system of observation and analysis imbibed in medical school, alongside the clinical practices developed in physicians' workday lives. They demonstrated what the aetiological, anatomical, and pathological presentation would look like for each disease, and re-constructed the experience of visiting a patient: the process of observation and treatment. The case history allowed the reader to experience as closely as possible what they might find in a real-life sick room and taught them how to make a correct diagnosis by showing them what it was important to know (Risse and Warner 1992; Riha 1995).

The case histories within psychiatric textbooks are interesting as they are cases chosen and edited for pedagogic value. These may not necessarily have been the most interesting or significant patients but were likely to have been those that the doctor considered as most illustrative or typical of the disease in question. They therefore represent an ideal of clinical practice and patient diagnosis. Jonathan Gillis has argued that these published case histories enable us to understand how doctors 'wanted the clinical encounter to be conducted and what they identified as the normative principles of practice to be passed on to medical students and other physicians' (Gillis 2006, p. 491). In the textbooks, practice is governed by the dominant psychiatric paradigm of the period: a physiological model of mental disease, rooted in anatomical-pathological knowledge. In the case of the female patient, this meant an epistemology of madness rooted in reproductive biology.

As a pedagogic tool, the case history needed to effectively impart an understanding of the treatment of mental disease and be meaningful for the reader. The textbook case history therefore performs an important role in communicating a legible (and learnable) version of each disorder, translated from theory to a 'real life' scenario. Making such complex information digestible is difficult. This was achieved through stripping away all the anomalies of clinical practice and maintaining similarity between individual cases histories, as well as between the written case and the actual experience of treating a patient. Familiarity was sustained through repetition of structural and lexical features as well as content, which produced a recognisable format. The cases in psychiatric textbooks followed the structure common to most published case histories in the second half of the nineteenth century and do this in three, interconnected ways: repetition of clinical signs, narrative structure, and authorial voice. These features were crucial in shaping clinical representations of female insanity as they directed what information doctors recorded about patients and, importantly, what significance was given to this data for the reader.

Firstly, specific signs of disease were repeated across multiple cases to highlight the most likely symptoms of insanity. Carol Berkenkotter (2008) argues that in psychiatry, clinical information is organised within the case history for diagnostic purposes. Linguistic and semantic devices 're-contextualise the patient's narrative of personal experience into a [...] framework that has been highly codified within the psychiatric profession' (Berkenkotter 2008, p. 2). Through analysing how the signs of mental illness have been codified, it is possible to better understand 'asylum doctors' perceptions of their patients, [and] the sense they made of their symptoms' (Berkenkotter 2008, p. 71). Case histories therefore reveal what signs of women's madness doctors thought it important to notice and can tell us about the interpretations given to these signs within the profession. In cases of female patients, psychiatric textbooks continually linked women's madness to uterine symptoms and sexual history. The repetition of these gendered signs of insanity across multiple case narratives imbued them with medical authority and reinforced a gendered understanding of the female mind.

Secondly, familiarity was maintained through the reproduction of a narrative structure which mimicked clinical practice, moving from consultation to observation to treatment plan. The clinical examination was retroactively separated into meaning-making categories: patient history, now loaded with etiological implications; observation, the truth spotting gaze of the physician; and treatment, the progress of disease organised into linear fashion to foreground clinical outcome. This ensured the reader was familiar with the process of consulting with a patient, and the attendant clinical methodology. It also told a story of disease, from sickness to cure, which supported the medical care of the insane (Rothfield 1995; Wright 2016). Jason Daniel Tougaw (2006) has explored the concurrent development of the realist novel and the case history, demonstrating (by highlighting similarities between both genres of writing) how storytelling is a fundamental feature of the nineteenth-century case. Tougaw suggests that 'to give individual cases the sense of an ending, physicians turned to the conventions of the novel,' providing closure through a complete narrative arc which compensated for the lack of 'epistemological certainty' provided by medical science itself (Tougaw 2006, p. 10). As Tougaw argues, the case history uses narrative to create an image of total truth. The organisation of female patients' disease histories within this narrative structure gave women's reproductive processes and behavioural patterns clinical significance, and made a theory grounded in female biology appear incontrovertible.

Lastly, the case histories were written in a passive clinical voice. This was designed to establish a standard of professional objectivity and interpret information gathered during the physician's examination in an ostensibly scientific manner. Meegan Kennedy has shown how the nineteenth-century medical case history embodies a 'clinical realism marked predominantly by mechanical objectivity' (Kennedy 2010, p. 4). Stemming from the profession's desire to exhibit 'accuracy and precision' in scientific knowledge and 'resist not only bias but judgement or any kind of mediation' (Kennedy 2010, p. 4) the tone of the case history was to approach as nearly as possible a 'disembodied, knowledgeable, and professional eye' (Kennedy 2010, p. 10). As Kennedy argues, the 'physician's affective relationship with the patient is obscured' in the production of a narrative voice which dispassionately reports on what is seen (Kennedy 2010, p. 58). Yet the self-abnegation of the author, through the attempted removal of the doctor-self from the narrative, is an illusion. Selection and judgement are always involved in the collection of facts. For example, case histories were rarely a verbatim record of what occurred in clinic. Patients' utterances were edited for sense, or strategically recontextualised in light of treatment outcomes. In cases of female insanity, this erased the personal experiences of the woman patient and reinforced the doctors' gendered perspective above any alternatives that may have been offered by the patient themselves. In addition, the clinical voice was maintained inconsistently, and the doctor's personal suppositions sometimes intrude on the clinical record.

Focusing on two of the most popular textbooks from the period, Bucknill and Tuke's *A Manual of Psychological Medicine* (1858) and William Bevan Lewis's *A Textbook of Mental Diseases* (1889), this chapter will now discuss how these features of the case history established a gendered model of female mental illness within psychiatry.

Case Histories and Gendered Signs of Mental Disease

To teach the reader how to diagnose different forms of insanity, textbook authors needed to write case histories that had continuity between multiple instances of the same disease. This would demonstrate how the disease would be likely to present itself and which symptoms commonly occurred. To aid physicians in noticing these symptoms (and making a correct diagnosis in a real-life clinical scenario), textbook authors repeated specific signs of disease across case histories. Bucknill and Tuke's hugely popular *Manual of Psychological Medicine* was the first of the textbooks to make a serious attempt at conveying clinical information in a structured manner and includes a 24-page appendix of cases. This appendix is split into three sections: cases showing types of insanity (to aid diagnosis); cases demonstrating good treatment; and cases demonstrating causation and pathology. Each case is classified into a particular diagnostic category (such as melancholia) and serves as an illustrative example of its class. Notably, case histories of female patients display a preoccupation with the reproductive functions, regardless of their diagnostic classification.

The first section of the appendix contains case histories corresponding to the frontispiece of the text, which includes several illustrations of insane patients, their physiognomies contorted into strange poses demonstrative of their condition (Fig. 2.2). These cases were intended to provide archetypal examples of different mental diseases. The uppermost portrait shows a woman looking somewhat mischievously out of the corner of her eyes. The appendix reveals hers to be a case of acute mania, labelled M. D., No. 1198. An 'excellent representation' of this type of insanity, the case outlines the woman's 'emotional and intellectual disturbance' (Bucknill and Tuke 1858, p. 507). Describing the patient and her history, the author remarks that she was once 'a remarkably handsome woman, and indeed still possesses the traces of her eminent beauty,' before ascribing the cause of her insanity to 'the birth of an illegitimate child' (Bucknill and Tuke 1858, p. 507). The doctor's physical examination of the patient covers the state of her health, her pulse and temperature, but also records that the 'functions of the uterus were normal' (Bucknill and Tuke 1858, p. 507). Even though the patient's disorder is not a specifically feminine disease, her reproductive history is clearly considered important. In the case of S. T., No. 1475, a forty-year-old woman with primary dementia, reproductive symptoms are equally as noteworthy. It is recorded in the description of the patient's symptoms that the 'catamenia [menstrual periods] are regular' (Bucknill and Tuke 1858, p. 510). The doctor also states that the woman was 'married to a shoemaker' and bore 'five children,' the youngest of whom 'she suckled to the date of her admission, affording an example of one means by which insanity is propagated' (Bucknill and Tuke 1858, p. 510).

In including the history and current state of the women's reproductive health, these clinical cases ascribe its significance in the diagnosis of insanity. Explicitly positioned as representative examples, the histories demonstrate to the reader how fundamental such symptoms are to female cases. They teach that the maternal life of the patient should be considered when searching for the origins of their illness and that the function of the reproductive system is of consequence in the progression of the disease. This remains the case in the *Manual*'s section on treatment methods, where female reproductive biology is significant not only from an aetiological, but a curative perspective.

Case A. C., No. 1641, described as 'Mania; recovery under emmenagogue treatment' suggests that menstruation both excited and cured a young girl's illness: emmenagogues are agents which bring on the menses (Bucknill and Tuke 1858, p. 517). The author notes that 'two months before admission, the catamenia became irregular, and mania supervened' (Bucknill and Tuke 1858, p. 517). He thus establishes a direct link between the girl's menstrual cycle, and her mental disease. Although it is not clear whether the catamenial irregularity is causal or symptomatic in nature, it exacerbates her instability: 'she was exceedingly violent, running

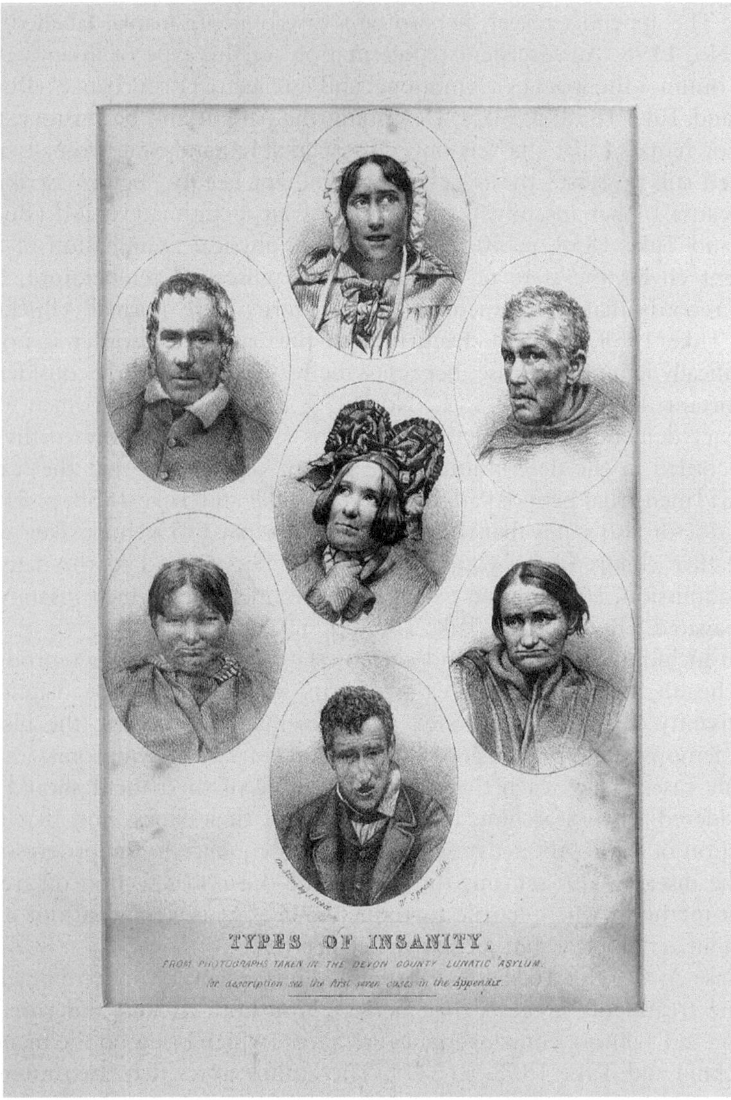

Fig. 2.2 'Types of Insanity', lithograph by W. Spread and J. Reed. Frontispiece to John Charles Bucknill and Daniel Hack Tuke. 1858. A Manual of Psychological Medicine: Containing the History, Nosology, Description, Statistics, Diagnosis, Pathology, and Treatment of Insanity, with an Appendix of Cases. London: John Churchill

round and round rooms and airing courts' (Bucknill and Tuke 1858, p. 517). Once admitted, she improved under treatment of 'warm baths, aperients, [and] muriate of morphia' (Bucknill and Tuke 1858, p. 517). Leeches to the groin were also applied but no cure was affected until the application of galvanism. 'The electro-galvanic current was passed across the pelvis for half an hour daily' and within two months 'this brought on the catamenia, and complete mental restoration followed' (Bucknill and Tuke 1858, p. 517). The appropriate treatment in this case was a regimen aimed at the menses, rather than the mental disorder directly, highlighting the close connection between menstrual and mental disturbance. The case history thus reinforces the sympathetic link between female reproductive organs and the mind, via the nerves, each having the power to influence the other.

These ideas had longevity within the profession. Published roughly thirty years after the first edition of the *Manual*, William Bevan Lewis's *A Textbook of Mental Diseases* was intended as an update to the classic text in 'light of recent research' (Bevan Lewis 1889, p. vii). The *Textbook* features case histories that are similar in content and purpose to those within the *Manual*, and the cases featuring women likewise operate under the same gendered assumptions. Bevan Lewis's *Textbook* reflected the changing landscape of psychiatry and included much greater detail on the anatomy and pathology of mental disease, towards which the attention of the profession had turned. The text is split into three parts accordingly: anatomy and histology; clinical findings; and pathology. The clinical section is divided into chapters which address diagnostic categories, such as puerperal insanity or states of depression. These are accompanied by case histories which he describes as 'typical illustrations' intended to demonstrate what might usually be met with in such patients (Bevan Lewis 1889, p. 140). As in the *Manual*, the cases covering types of female insanity foreground the reproductive history and symptoms of the patient, positioning them as integral to the disease. Despite advancements in scientific practice, Bevan Lewis draws many of the same conclusions as his colleagues, Bucknill and Tuke.

In the chapter on climacteric insanity (insanity of menopause), Bevan Lewis describes the case of S. H., a forty-two-year-old married woman. The woman had strong suicidal tendencies and was very depressed. Having been 'consistent and temperate' prior to her admission, the sole cause of her insanity is given as the cessation of her menstrual cycle (Bevan

Lewis 1889, p. 394). He notes that she was 'suffering from the functional ailments incident to the menstrual climacteric' and that 'she had been melancholic' for three months (Bevan Lewis 1889, p. 394). The 'catamenia were arrested' and had been for around eight months prior to her admission (Bevan Lewis 1889, p. 394). The next case history describes another woman with the same disorder, forty-seven-year-old A. A. However, this patient exhibited different symptoms. Admitted in a 'state of subacute excitement,' she is described as 'dangerously aggressive' (Bevan Lewis 1889, p. 395). Suffering from maniacal attacks and delusions, the patient is the opposite of the previous case. Despite this, the aetiology of her illness is described almost identically: prior to the onset of insanity, she was 'steady' and 'temperate,' and was also 'at the menopause' (Bevan Lewis 1889, p. 395). In both cases Bevan Lewis identifies the reproductive symptoms of the patient as the defining feature of the disease. Even if the presentation is dissimilar, if the patient is undergoing menopause, then the disease is nosologically identical. Diagnosis rests not on psychological or behavioural manifestations of lunacy but on the uterine irregularity considered to be at the heart of the illness.

The clinical case history therefore gave special etiological or pathological significance to reproductive symptoms in women and consequently assigned an excitatory or curative role to changes in a woman's reproductive health, both from a physiological and social perspective (Table 2.3). These gendered signs formed a language of diagnosis common to all female cases: reproductive symptoms in women were not indicative of specific mental diseases but were symbolic of a peculiar feminine derangement. It is the repetition and reproduction of these gendered signs across all classes of insanity which constructs a theory of women's madness that links female reproductive health, through the nervous system, to brain functioning and thus to mental disease.

The preoccupation with a woman's reproductive functions arose out of the gendered preconceptions which doctors brought to their consultations with female patients. Mind doctors approached the case from within a culture which saw motherhood and the ability to reproduce as integral to womanhood. Combining a physiological model of insanity with social ideologies of gender, the authors gave women's reproductive health primary importance in the origins of female madness. At a time when the profession was struggling for legitimacy as a medical field, mind doctors looked for physical signs of disease in the body as evidence of the disordered mental processes which they did not fully understand. Seeing the

Table 2.3 Clinical signs relevant to female madness in psychiatric textbook case histories, 1845–1895

Physiological signs	*Social signs*
• Childbearing history	• Marital status
- Number of children	• Domestic strife
- Recent or current pregnancies	• Erotic behaviour (often a secondary symptom of uterine disturbance)
- Illegitimate births	
- Difficult births	• Unfeminine behaviour
• Lactation and breastfeeding	- Aggressiveness
• Regularity of menstruation	- Loudness
• Entering the climacteric	- Restlessness
• Ovarian or uterine health	- Excitability or irritability
- Irritation	
- Cysts	
- Leucorrhoea	
- Lochia	

male body as the default human form, the reproductive differences so apparent in the female body appeared to be signs of disruption. Through their use as an educational tool these case histories taught students and practitioners that reproductive and sexual symptoms were important to look for in women patients.

Although the perpetuation of gendered ideologies in Victorian society can only be explained by the examination of several complex factors, the medicalisation of these beliefs within textbooks no doubt contributed to their authority. The case history was crucial to this process through its semantic positioning of female reproduction as clinically significant information, thereby transforming cultural beliefs into medical evidence; a transformation which imbued such beliefs with validity and permanency.

Case Narrative and Gendered Clinical Practice

A gendered approach to the female mind was also facilitated by the form of the case history. Designed to teach a diagnostic methodology, the narrative structure of the case history is formulaic, with each case divided into sections dealing with a stage of the treatment process: the patient examination, during which the disease history is given and observations are made on current symptoms; the treatment itself, unfolding over days or weeks with variations or improvements noted; and outcome, usually cure as the treatment plan described was intended to demonstrate the correct methodology. These categories had an instructional value, demonstrating what the reader should do when encountering an insane patient. They also held an analytic purpose, as organising information into these discrete stages gave clinical significance to what was recorded. The placement of gendered signs of madness at specific moments in the narrative of the case therefore gave them particular meaning. The recording of a patient's menstruation, for example, might have an entirely different emphasis whether it was noted in the symptoms or outcome portion of the history.

In the case histories from both the *Textbook* and *Manual* these gendered signs (such as the interruption of the menses or a recent birth) are often included in the section on disease history and patient examination, which gave them aetiological significance. Bucknill and Tuke's case G. N., No. 588 gives the climacteric period as a cause of suicidal melancholia (Bucknill and Tuke 1858, pp. 514–516). Case M. A., No. 1707 notes desertion by the husband as a catalyst for insanity, with leucorrhoea and uterine irritation as symptoms (Bucknill and Tuke 1858, p. 517). Bevan Lewis frequently discusses the importance of noticing reproductive changes in female cases, describing their 'complex nature' and stressing that they could either be 'the *cause* of a mental storm' or 'a symptom of associated arrest in the development of the central nervous system' (Bevan Lewis 1889, p. 374).

In his *Textbook*, Bevan Lewis writes of the case of A. H., a nineteen-year-old housemaid suffering from ovarian derangement and mania. Describing the history of the patient he notes that 'she exhibited no eccentricity prior to the attack' and was of 'good moral character,' the only significant change being that 'for a considerable period the catamenia had been suppressed' (Bevan Lewis 1889, p. 347). He thus introduces the idea that menstrual irregularity may be important in the case. Next, in his examination of the patient, he records that her behaviour was 'utterly regardless of decency,' her 'excitement was intense,' and she was 'garrulous,' 'flighty, sudden, and impulsive' (Bevan Lewis 1889, p. 347). We therefore learn that her symptoms are manic and sexually indecent in nature and are probably linked to her menstrual problems in some way. Bevan Lewis then outlines the progress of her treatment. At first 'an aloetic purge was ordered' alongside 'phosphate of iron' (Bevan Lewis 1889, p. 347). There was 'decided improvement' in her mood and behaviour, but the patient still complained of pain in the abdomen and lumbar region (Bevan Lewis 1889, p. 347). Bevan Lewis writes that 'these symptoms were apparently due to congestion of the [spinal] cord and its membranes from suppressed menstrual flow,' clinical observations confirming the suspicions aroused in the first part of the case (Bevan Lewis 1889, p. 347). Once this decision had been made, he altered her treatment and ordered spinal douches as well as iron. This began to work, and 'in three months from admission' the patient was much more 'self-controlled' (Bevan Lewis 1889, p. 347). He finally records the outcome of the case: 'the catamenial flow was re-established coincident with the greatly improved health, the spinal symptoms referable thereto disappeared, and the patient was discharged recovered' (Bevan Lewis 1889, p. 347).

The case history unravels the progress of the housemaid's illness piece by piece, eventually revealing that the patient's suppressed menstruation was acting upon her nervous system via the spinal cord and producing mental derangement. The first observations of the absence of the catamenia and indecent behaviour have etiological and diagnostic significance in relation to the final classification of the patient's disease. The case narrative unfolds these events just as if the reader were experiencing it first-hand and reacting to the information he gathered in the clinical setting. This pretence of real-time observation replicated the treatment process, although of course the author had prior knowledge of the case in its totality. Bevan Lewis thus used the narrative structure of the case history to fashion the housemaid's illness into a coherent story of disease where reproductive symptoms are pivotal factors in the progression of the case.

Peter Brooks' (1992) work on plot is useful here for understanding how narrative structure shapes this information. Brooks defines plot as the 'design and intention of narrative, what shapes a story and gives it a certain direction or intent of meaning' (Brooks 1992, p. xi). It is the 'principle of interconnectedness' that allows us to move progressively through discrete elements of the narrative (Brooks 1992, p. 4–5). This progressive movement is key to the nature of plot, which functions as a 'dynamic shaping force' and is 'goal-oriented and forward moving' (Brooks 1992, pp. 12–13). Plot therefore enables the telling of stories through its ability to produce cognitive and semantic links between events. In the case history, the plot makes sense of the myriad observations made by the physician. The formalised narrative structure of the history allows this plot to progress through time from an etiological origin, through the intervention of treatment, to a conclusion of patient recovery (or death). This, as Brooks has described, is the 'necessary retrospectivity of narrative: that only the end can finally determine meaning' (Brooks 1992, p. 22).

Case histories are not a neutral reflection of events at the clinic or asylum. The act of writing a case history is an after-the-fact ordering of events; the author has intervened between event and page to turn clinical experience into an orderly narrative. The published form we read in the textbook is a rewriting, not only of this experience but also some earlier form of case notes made on scene and kept in the patient casebook. Such rewriting has been done with a pedagogic purpose in mind; the case histories were deliberately selected (and perhaps even adapted) to teach the reader something specific about insanity. It is through the arrangement of clinical information into a linear story of disease and cure that the case history performs its didactic function.

The case of M. A., No. 1707, in Bucknill and Tuke's *Manual*, is a particularly good example of the effects of plot on the retelling of patient history. The case describes a female patient suffering from mania and irregular uterine function, specifically 'profuse leucorrhoea [vaginal discharge]' (Bucknill and Tuke 1858, p. 517). Treatment was pharmacological, the patient being administered several different drugs which were injected into her vagina twice daily. This 'succeeded in stopping the leucorrhoea' and she was discharged 'in good health, three months after admission' (Bucknill and Tuke 1858, p. 517). This case history positions uterine symptoms as a cause of mental disease and a return to regular gynaecological function has a direct impact upon the patient's insanity. However, this is an artificial narrative progression. The case history includes only the data which the doctor-author decided pertained to the patient's disorder. The process of writing clinical cases was selective, editing anything extraneous that the patient may have said or done. We hear little of the mental symptoms the woman might have experienced, or of the emotional or social factors at play in the history of her disease. Her gynaecological problems are spotlighted as signs of sickness and followed through with focused treatment. This produces a rather narrow approach to female madness; the lesson being that a doctor should always search for such symptoms and act upon them if found.

Despite this obvious reworking, the psychiatric case history represented an ideal of clinical objectivity and insight. In textbooks particularly, they are a distillation of knowledge, edited and organised to present a consensus on mental disease that would be learnable and repeatable in the reader's own practice. Utilised as an educational tool, the case history taught the student or physician about methodologies of clinical practice in the mind sciences and how to make sense out of the data gathered through such practices. As Tougaw (2006) has shown, the narrative structure of the case history transformed the chaos of random observations into a meaningful clinical story. In cases of women's madness, this process created a trajectory that linked reproductive symptoms or deviant sexual behaviour to lunacy.

The Clinical Voice and the Erasure of Female Experience

Important to the structure of the case history was the voice of the narrator themselves, the doctor-author, who directed the reader to pertinent observations and moved the narrative onwards. This clinical voice was detached and analytic, which gave to the conclusions recorded an empiric appearance. However, an examination of this technique can uncover how the doctors' ostensibly objective descriptions were in reality shaped by the cultural and social preconceptions they inevitably brought to bear on any patient examination. As mentioned, the narrator records only the observations which they deem necessary to demonstrate correct diagnosis. The case histories thus often discard the personal testimony of the patient or subsume it within the physician's retroactive analysis of what occurred. Yet the case history disguises this. The doctor-author's account appears neutral, and the facts of the case often seem complete. It is only when read against the grain that these case histories can be revealed as interpretation and selection rather than passive observation.

Carol Berkenkotter (2008) warns that even when the words of the subject are reported in case histories, we should be wary of assuming that they are a verbatim account, as authors tended to recontextualise what the patient said to demonstrate clinical significance to the reader. She argues that this results in what she terms a double narrative, in which the physician and patient stories exist simultaneously within the case history. This 'narrative-within-a-narrative is noteworthy because of the linguistic and semantic devices the therapist uses,' recoding the personal into the clinical (Berkenkotter 2008, p. 2). Case histories within the textbooks perform this restructuring of patient experience. Although they do so for both male and female patients, the cases featuring women subjects are particularly interesting in revealing how specifically female experiences or behaviours were coded with pathological import. The dominance of the clinical voice (viewed as objective and scientific), over first-hand descriptions of mental disease (viewed as subjective and personal), re-presented feminine behaviours or life experiences within a pathological framework which supported a gendered theory of female mental illness.

As was common in clinical case histories, the patients in both the *Manual* and *Textbook* remain nameless, identified only by their initials and a short description giving their age and occupational or marital status. This lack of personal identification creates a disconnect between the reader and the patient, divesting the sick of their personhood by focusing solely on their disease. Intended to preserve the privacy of the subject, this anonymity yet serves to erase the patient. In cases which give the history of female lunatics, often the first thing the reader learns about the patient is whether she is a wife or mother. In Bevan Lewis's text, M. A. W. is identified as a 'married woman with a family of two children,' and M. A. H is 'single, a young girl of delicate physique' (Bevan Lewis 1889, p. 340). S. M. was 'married twelve months ago, and delivered of her first child three months before her admission' (Bevan Lewis 1889, p. 381). The positioning of such biographical details at the start of the narrative—often with extremely little other personal information to go on—reinforces the clinical importance of these domestic experiences at the expense of other life events. In recording occupational and marital status, women's role in the home is highlighted. Conversely, the cases concerning male patients, whilst stating employment, do not always record whether the man has a family.

The sense of the patient as a diagnostic subject is sustained throughout the case history by the use of third person narration and hearsay testimony when describing patients' symptoms. German Berrios (1996) has shown how, during the nineteenth century, a patient's internal experiences were seen as a legitimate field of inquiry for the first time. The patient's complaints, ideas or descriptions of their feelings became clinical observations which served as evidence of mental disease, and dialogue between patient and physician was a key part of the examination process. The purpose of the dialogue was not to understand the first-hand experiences of the sufferer as closely as possible but to gather information to aid in diagnosis. The patients are certainly treated this way in the textbooks, where the insane person's experiences are recorded second-hand by the physician, or even third-hand through the physician's record of the remarks of a patient's friends and family. The case of M. P., No. 1691, from Bucknill and Tuke's *Manual*, covers a woman suffering from 'acute mania from moral causes' and records her delusions (Bucknill and Tuke 1858, p. 518). The doctor writes that she 'says her body and soul are lost, that she shall be burned alive, that she sees hell flames, that she cannot be cured' (Bucknill and Tuke 1858, p. 518). Reported in the third person, we lose the sense of the patient's voice and of the distress which must have accompanied these words. This distancing renders such statements impersonal. They become relevant only for their diagnostic significance and for the relationship which they demonstrate between the content of the delusions and her immoral act, 'adultery with a married man' (Bucknill and Tuke 1858, p. 518).

Similarly, in the case of M. W. from Bevan Lewis' *Textbook*, a thirty-nine-year-old woman diagnosed with lactational insanity, we hear of her feelings only through the doctor's shorthand report of their conversations. Although he writes that 'she was communicative upon admission, and discoursed readily upon the subject of her mental ailments,' Bevan Lewis does not record what the woman said (Bevan Lewis 1889, p. 378). Instead, he describes the patient's symptoms second-hand: 'her health began to fail, [then] restlessness, low spirits, suicidal feelings' all ensued (Bevan Lewis 1889, p. 378). He notes that 'ever since weaning the child she had been depressed' and that she had 'found her memory impaired of late and this had troubled her greatly' (Bevan Lewis 1889, p. 378). The sense of dialogue between the patient and practitioner has all but disappeared and the case history completely disguises the process of selection involved in the clinical examination. In writing up his notes from the interview, Bevan Lewis recorded the remarks he considered useful for the treatment of the case, whilst presenting his discourse as passive observation. What the reader has access to in the published version is his interpretation of their conversation, reconfigured as medical facts. This not only causes a loss of much of the patient's personal experience and agency, it also effaces the methods by which such information is gained. It is unclear whether the feelings the woman describes are those which she revealed during free discourse, or whether (as is more likely) Bevan Lewis led her to express them during questioning.

Significantly, the case history impresses the reader with the sympathetic link between the patient's experiences as a new, breastfeeding mother and the negative feelings she expresses. She had 'brought up the infant at the breast until four months since, when depression supervened,' and had been 'frequently tempted to injure herself' since ceasing to feed the child

(Bevan Lewis 1889, p. 378). It is unclear whether the emphasis on breast-feeding in the woman's insanity is made by the doctor or the patient. During examination, the dialogue would have been guided by the physician's theories. The questions he might ask a female patient were thus directed by prevailing assumptions about the etiological role of reproduction in women's madness. A report of such a dialogue, as is recorded in the case history of M. W., would highlight the significance of these questions to the reader, apparently through the utterances of the patient herself.

It is difficult to unpack where and how the doctor has interpreted or directed the patient's words because of the apparent objectivity of the clinical voice and its consistency across different case histories. However, the final section of cases in the *Manual* (on the pathology of mental disease) contains revealing afterthoughts. These cases were intended to teach the reader about changes caused in the brain by disease and describe patients who have died in the asylum. They therefore include post-mortem notes in addition to the main body of the case history. Interestingly, perhaps because of the lack of conclusive evidence such research offered during the nineteenth century, a number of these notes finish with the personal surmises of the writer. In cases of female patients, these remarks demonstrate how the doctors' attitude to mental disease in women was influenced by social and cultural prejudices.

In the case of A. V., No. 579, a patient suffering from 'Monomania, with Religious Exaltation, of long standing,' is recorded as having died of an ulcer unrelated to her mental condition (Bucknill and Tuke 1858, p. 522). The case history notes that she was 'unmarried, aged fifty-three' and that the primary symptoms of her insanity were a tendency to 'religious enthusiasm' and to lecture others on theological matters in a 'loud, pertinacious manner' (Bucknill and Tuke 1858, p. 522). She lived in the asylum for a number of years and never recovered. After noting the outcome of the post-mortem, the author writes:

'The case affords an example of the slight deviations from the normal state which take place in cases of emotional monomania, or moral insanity, which arise from exaggeration of the natural disposition. This patient was only some degrees removed from those offensive preaching women one occasionally meets with in society. Probably marriage and the cares of a family would have saved her from an asylum. What, in this country, can a single woman do, with an energetic brain weighing more than three pounds, but get into some trouble or other' (Bucknill and Tuke 1858, p. 523)?

This rather bizarre mixture of anatomical evidence and social commentary reveals the slippage between the cultural assumptions of the writer and his scientific conclusions. The patient is placed on a sliding scale of irritating female behaviour, predictable in spinsters who have devoted their energies to religion rather than a family. In this case, the patient's spinsterhood has become pathological. The suggestion that this could have been avoided if the patient had only married demonstrates the importance given to domestic and maternal activities in preserving female health through their role as the proper object of feminine desire. Woman's cherished place in the home, integral to Victorian social harmony, is given physiological significance. The consequence of avoiding this natural outlet is an accumulation of superfluous and implicitly sexual energy, potentially leading to insanity.

The next case history in the textbook features a patient who is unable to control these sexual feelings. The patient, J. M, was a thirty-year-old woman with 'Acute Nymphomania' accompanied by suicidal impulses (Bucknill and Tuke 1858, p. 523). Stating that she had previously had attacks of mania, the author notes that 'no cause could be assigned' to the appearance of the new symptoms. She had apparently randomly entered a parish church and, 'during divine service, thrown herself prostrate upon the pavement and made a scene' (Bucknill and Tuke 1858, p. 523). Once admitted, the patient 'made a violent and indecent attack on a woman she believed to be a man' and 'constant attacks of an indecent nature' upon her nurses (Bucknill and Tuke 1858, pp. 523–524). These attacks were interspersed with many attempts at suicide and self-harm, and the author records that the patient 'evidently suffered great mental anguish' (Bucknill and Tuke, p. 524). She died of asthenia (weakness) shortly after arrival. The author comments on her case:

'This poor young woman bore an exemplary moral character, directly at variance from that which might physiologically have been expected from the indications offered by her conformation and temperament. Vehement mental perturbation appears to have resulted from the struggle between mental purity and the physiological impulses of sex. The acute cerebral hyperaemia was sympathetic with the state of the ovaries, and affords an illustration of the conditions of the brain in sympathetic disturbance' (Bucknill and Tuke 1858, p. 524).

The doctor's compassion for the young woman, so obviously feeling enormous shame for her conduct, arises out of his conviction that her pure intentions are at war with her bodily, sexual impulses. These impulses are uncontrollable and dirty, in contrast with the female mind which is moral and chaste. The tragedy of the female body is its innate sexuality, which the conscious mind must always regulate. In cases of sexual insanity, this regulatory power is lost, and passionate urges force themselves to the surface. The morbid state of the ovaries and brain is given as the cause of this type of insanity, thus providing clinical evidence for the patient's inability to supress these feelings. However, if we re-read the case from a socio-cultural perspective, we can understand the woman's anguish as a very real guilt for feelings of sexual desire, a taboo which was rigorously policed in Victorian society through narratives of the fallen woman and legislation designed to punish those sexually active outside of marriage.

In both cases culturally significant female behaviours are reconfigured as evidence of insanity. These behaviours serve as barometers of mental health by measuring the degree to which the patient was able to act appropriately. The women's diagnoses were based on their inability to behave modestly and submissively. These examples thus reveal how gendered social ideologies influenced clinical practice. Eliding patient experiences with their own observations to present a clinically focused view of their case, the doctor-narrator appears objective. Closer examination, however, reveals socio-cultural influences which complicate these assumptions. It is thus necessary, when reading the case histories in psychiatric textbooks, to keep sight of the clinical voice as an active contextualising force, writing from within a patriarchal value system which informed a gendered epistemology of female madness.

Conclusion

The genre of the psychiatric textbook emerged in the mid-nineteenth century in response to the lack of formalised education available in the mind sciences. The textbooks were practical guides which aimed to fill this gap in clinical knowledge. Proving popular, they became the primary way in which physicians learnt about the discipline, the theories of mind which they contained becoming the dominant paradigm of insanity in the second half of the nineteenth century. These textbooks established a gendered concept of female insanity based in cultural beliefs about women's maternal and domestic role in society, which highlighted reproductive symptoms in mentally ill women. The textbooks thus medicalised social ideologies of gender, reproducing them as clinical facts and demonstrating their application in psychiatric practice. Psychiatric textbooks, and the literary techniques which they deployed as pedagogic tools, were therefore instrumental in the development and communication of nineteenth-century theories of female insanity within the medical profession.

The use of clinical case histories as an educational tool was integral to this process. They reinforced a gendered theory of disease through the repetition of reproductive diagnostic signs across multiple cases; through the organisation of patients' disease histories within a narrative structure which gave women's behaviour and reproductive processes clinical significance; and through the use of a clinical voice which completely elided female experiences of mental illness. Contrary to Andrew Scull's (1979) claims, the case notes kept meticulously by asylum staff were not simply time-filling, bureaucratic record keeping, but a way to collate knowledge and make sense of clinical observations. They were essential to the enterprise of psychiatry.

This chapter thus explains how the combination of three factors—the physiological model of insanity, social ideologies of gender, and the professionalisation of the mind sciences—influenced the formation of psychiatric theories about women's minds. It also builds on the work of Elaine Showalter (1987) and other feminist historians of psychiatry to locate the site of this formation in written discourse. This is not the end of the story, however. These theories did not remain static within psychiatric textbooks, but were read, adopted, communicated, and challenged beyond their pages. The next chapter moves beyond medical literature to investigate how medical theories about women's minds changed as they entered the public realm and how they came, full circle, to impact cultural beliefs about femininity.

References

Unpublished Sources

Author's Ledgers. 1845–1900. Archive of the House of Longman, Churchill. Microfilms 57–62.

Catalogue of the Central Lending Library. 1894. Leeds Central Library Archive. MS L017.1 LEE.

Catalogue of the Joint Library of the Medical Department of the Yorkshire College and the Leeds and West-Riding Medico-Chirurgical Society. 1892. University of Leeds Archive. ACA/001/BOX 9.

Merkulova, Polina. 2016. The Making of a Manual: A History of the Classic Textbook of Victorian Psychiatry. MA dissertation, University of Leeds.

Published Sources

Altick, Richard D. 1999. Publishing. In *A Companion to Victorian Literature and Culture*, ed. Herbert F. Tucker, 289–304. Oxford: Blackwell.

Andrews, Jonathan. 1998. Documents and Sources: Case Notes, Case Histories, and the Patient's Experience of Insanity at Gartnavel Royal Asylum, Glasgow, in the Nineteenth Century. *Social History of Medicine* 11: 255–281. https://doi.org/10.1093/shm/11.2.255.

Benignus Winslow, Forbes. 1860. *On Obscure Diseases of the Brain and Disorders of the Mind*. London: Churchill.

Berkenkotter, Carol. 2008. *Patient Tales: Case Histories and the Uses of Narrative in Psychiatry*. Hampton: University of South Carolina Press.

Berrios. German E. 1996. *The History of Mental Symptoms: Descriptive Psychopathology Since the Nineteenth Century*. Cambridge: Cambridge University Press.

Bevan Lewis, William. 1889. *A Textbook of Mental Diseases*. London: Charles Griffin.

Beveridge, Allan. 1991. Thomas Clouston and the Edinburgh School of Psychiatry. In *150 Years of British Psychiatry: 1841–1991*, ed. German E. Berrios and Hugh Freeman, 359–366. London: Gaskell.

Beveridge, Allan. 1998. The Odd Couple: The Partnership of J. C. Bucknill and D. H. Tuke. *Psychiatric Bulletin*. 22: 52–56. https://doi.org/10.1192/pb.22.1.52.

Bonner, Thomas Neville. 2000. *Becoming a Physician: Medical Education in Britain, France, Germany, and the United States, 1750–1945*. Baltimore: John Hopkins University Press.

Brooks, Peter. 1992. *Reading for the Plot: Design and Intention in Narrative*. Cambridge: Harvard University Press.

Bucknill, John Charles, and Daniel Hack Tuke. 1858. *A Manual of Psychological Medicine: The History, Nosology, Description, Statistics, Diagnosis, Pathology, and Treatment of Insanity, with an Appendix of Cases*. London: John Churchill.

Bynum, William F. 1991. Tuke's *Dictionary* and Psychiatry at the Turn of the Century. In *150 Years of British Psychiatry: 1841–1991*, ed. German E. Berrios and Hugh Freeman, 163–179. London: Gaskell.

Catalogue of Books in the Medical and Biological Libraries at University College London. 1887. London: Taylor and Francis.

Crichton Browne, James. 1861. *The Clinical Teaching of Psychology: A Valedictory Address*. Edinburgh: James Nichol.

Csiszar, Alex. 2018. *Authorship and the Politics of Knowledge in the Nineteenth Century*. Chicago: Chicago University Press.

Eliot, Simon. 2000. The Business of Victorian Publishing. In *The Cambridge Companion to the Victorian Novel*, ed. Deirdre David, 37–60. Cambridge: Cambridge University Press.

Eliot, Simon. 2009. From Few and Expensive to Many and Cheap: The British Book Market 1800–1890. In *A Companion to the History of the Book*, ed. Simon Eliot and Jonathan Rose, 291–302. Oxford: Wiley-Blackwell.

Fielding Blandford, George. 1871. *Insanity and its Treatment; Lectures on the Treatment, Medical and Legal, of Insane Patients*. Edinburgh: Oliver and Boyd.

Foucault, Michel. 2003. *The Birth of the Clinic: An Archaeology of Medical Perception,* trans. by A. M. Sheridan. Abingdon: Routledge.

Gillis, Jonathan. 2006. The History of the Patient History Since 1850. *Bulletin of the History of Medicine* 80: 490–512. https://doi.org/10.1353/bhm.2006.0097.

Hagberg Wright, C. T. 1909. *The Subject-Index of the London Library, St James's Square, London*. London: Williams and Northgate.

Hyslop, Theo B. 1895. *Mental Physiology: Especially in its Relations to Mental Disorders*. London: J & A Churchill.

Kennedy, Meegan. 2010. *Vision and Representation in Victorian Medical Narrative and the Novel*. Athens: Ohio University Press.

Malane, Rachel. 2005. *Sex in Mind: The Gendered Brain in Nineteenth-Century Literature and Mental Sciences*. New York: Peter Lang.

Marland, Hilary. 2004. *Dangerous Motherhood: Insanity and Childbirth in Victorian Britain*. Basingstoke: Palgrave Macmillan.

Medical Books: *A Manual of Psychological Medicine*. 1859. *Athenaeum*. 1632: 192.

Physiology, Mental. 1897. Especially in its Relations to Mental Disorders. *Journal of Mental Science* 43: 150–152.

Noble, Daniel. 1853. *Elements of Psychological Medicine: An Introduction to the Practical Study of Insanity, Adapted for Students and General Practitioners*. London: John Churchill.

On Obscure Diseases of the Brain and Disorders of the Mind, their Incipient Symptoms, Pathology, Diagnosis, Treatment and Prophylaxis. 1860. *Edinburgh Review*. 112: 526–545.

Porter, Roy. 1999. *The Greatest Benefit to Mankind: A Medical History of Humanity from Antiquity to the Present*. London: Fontana.

Riha, Ortun. 1995. Surgical Case Records as an Historical Source: Limits and Perspectives. *Social History of Medicine*. 8: 271–283. https://doi.org/10.1093/shm/8.2.271.

Risse, Guenter B., and Harley Warner. 1992. Reconstructing Clinical Activities: Patient Records in Medical History. *Social History of Medicine*. 5: 183–205. https://doi.org/10.1093/shm/5.2.183.

Rothfield, Lawrence. 1995. *Vital Signs: Medical Realism in Nineteenth-Century Fiction*. Princeton: Princeton University Press.

Royal College of Physicians of London. 1912. *Catalogue of the Library*. London: Spottiswoode and Co.

Savage, George Henry. 1884. *Insanity and Allied Neuroses: Practical and Clinical*. London: Cassell & Co.

Secord, James A. 2003. *Victorian Sensation: The Extraordinary Publication, Reception, and Secret Authorship of Vestiges of the Natural History of Creation*. Chicago: University of Chicago Press.

Scull, Andrews. 1979. *Museums of Madness: The Social Organisation of Insanity in Nineteenth-Century England*. London: Allen Lane.

Showalter, Elaine. 1987. *The Female Malady: Women, Madness, and English Culture, 1830–1980*. London: Virago.

Smith Clouston, Thomas. 1883. *Clinical Lectures on Mental Diseases*. London: J & A Churchill.

St. Clair, William. 2004. *The Reading Nation in the Romantic Period*. Cambridge: Cambridge University Press.

Tougaw, Jason Daniel. 2006. *Strange Cases: The Medical Case History and the British Novel*. Abingdon: Routledge.

Weedon, Alexis. 2003. *Victorian Publishing: The Economics of Book Production for a Mass Market, 1836–1916*. Aldershot: Ashgate.

Williams, Joseph. 1852. *Insanity, its Causes, Prevention, and Cure: Including Apoplexy, Epilepsy, and Congestion of the Brain*. London: John Churchill.

Wright, David. 1998. The Certification of Insanity in Nineteenth-Century England and Wales. *History of Psychiatry* 9: 267–290. https://doi.org/10.1177/0957154X9800903501.

Wright, Erika. 2016. *Reading for Health: Medical Narratives and the Nineteenth-Century Novel*. Athens: Ohio University Press.

CHAPTER 3

The Female Mind in the Periodical Press: Henry Maudsley and the Sociological Application of Gendered Psychiatric Theory

Nineteenth-century mind doctors believed the female body was at the mercy of a reproductive system which made women uniquely vulnerable to the kinds of nervous irritation that would produce mental disease. As the previous chapter has shown, this theory was well established in textbooks for the alienist and wider medical community. In addition to these textbooks, specialist periodicals established a shared literature for those working in the care of the insane. Publications such as the Medico-Psychological Association's *Journal of Mental Science* (1858–1962) published interesting case histories and articles by doctors putting forward their latest theories on the mind. These journals, which were essential for professional advancement and communication, likewise relied on this core belief about the pathology of female nature and reinforced a gendered concept of women's mental instability.

Such literature was designed for a specialist audience of asylum physicians and other medical men and in practice was not widely read beyond this community. Yet this image of the female mind as essentially unsound found its way beyond the boundaries of the scientific press and appeared in the pages of non-specialist and popular periodicals. In the latter half of the nineteenth century, many articles, essays, gossip columns, news pieces, court reports, literary representations, illustrations and other forms of printed matter discussed mental disease in women didactically,

M. Chapman, *Writing Women's Madness, 1845–1914*, Palgrave Studies in Literature, Science and Medicine,
https://doi.org/10.1007/978-3-031-97092-4_3

discursively, and colloquially. This content appeared across a range of publications in different price brackets, including quarterlies, the new monthly reviews, and weeklies.[1] Significantly, this cacophony of voices did not merely report what mind doctors thought; public discourse on the female mind was both active and transformative.

This was in part due to the range of authorships permissible within the periodical genre. One did not have to be a mind doctor to write and publish on the mind, and those doctors who did write articles on female mental disease were often not specialists in the mind sciences. In fact, many individuals without medical training of any kind contributed to discussions on insanity in general periodicals. The developing nature of the mind sciences during the nineteenth century resulted in a lack of professional visibility in the press, creating space for other forms of authority on the female mind to take centre stage. Moreover, medical theories could be applied for different purposes. Information about the female mind was imparted in non-specialist journals not to improve clinical expertise but to entertain, inform, or support arguments about public concerns. These changes in both textual form and audience (from textbook to gossip column and from mind doctors to members of the public) allowed alternative ideas of the female mind to take shape. Non-specialist periodicals, accommodating different generic parameters to clinical writing, enabled professional theories not only to be read but also reproduced and, crucially, challenged by those outside of the alienist community.

This chapter will explore one example from the popular press, which is representative of this discursive shift: the publication of Henry Maudsley's 'Sex in Mind and in Education' in the April 1874 number of the *Fortnightly Review*, and the debate that followed. Maudsley applied his clinical theories on the female mind to the social question of higher education for women, arguing that serious study made girls prone to nervous illness. Several critics, such as Joan Burstyn (1980), Elaine Showalter (1987), and Katharina Rowold (2011), have thus placed the essay in the context of both female emancipation and the mind sciences in the late nineteenth century, demonstrating that Maudsley utilised gendered medical theories

[1] In the ProQuest British Periodicals database, there are numerous hits for articles related to women's madness published between 1845 and 1895. For example, a search for 'hysteria' generates over 1000 results. Combining the terms 'female', 'brain', and 'insanity' generates a further 2000, 'insanity and pregnancy' a trimmer 220.

to justify the continuation of women's inferior position in society. Yet these studies have neglected to address the significance of the article's publication in a non-specialist periodical and the ripples of impact that spread through the press as readers responded to Maudsley's theories. The controversy caused by the article's topic sparked a lively debate that continued for weeks after its appearance. This debate came at a turning point in female education, as women began to gain access to universities and to medical training. The letters and essays written in reply to Maudsley are thus an unexamined part of women's history.

'Sex in Mind and in Education' is an important essay for two reasons. Firstly, the article is a rare example of a mind doctor writing directly to a lay audience. Although plenty of content on insanity was published in general periodicals this was not often authored by professionals in the mind sciences, who tended to produce specialist literature for an equally specialist audience. Maudsley's essay is unusual in that, crossing this boundary, it addresses a social problem from a medical perspective. In doing so, his article exposes the circular logic in the relationship between psychiatric theories of the female mind and nineteenth-century gender ideologies. Secondly, the debate following the publication of his essay demonstrated how Maudsley's ideas could be adapted in support of diverse viewpoints. The essay's distinctive combination of medical authorship, socially relevant subject matter, and readerly accessibility meant that psychiatric theories of the female mind were left open for interpretation and dispute. Crucially, the discussion of Maudsley's article in non-specialist periodicals enabled women to have their views heard as, unlike the medical journals of the time, these publications were open to submissions from female authors. The range of textual genres available to writers facilitated this diversity of responses in the press.

This chapter will first consider what kind of content was being published on mental disease in the popular press at this time, and how 'Sex in Mind and in Education' fitted within this context. It will then discuss the significance of the article's publication, both for Maudsley and for the psychiatric profession as a whole, before examining his ideas on the female mind and the rebuttals to his article. Maudsley's foray into the public press came at an exciting moment in the development of professional and public discourses about the nature of the female mind and is a useful source for understanding the complex intersection of cultural and medical beliefs about the female brain in the mid nineteenth century.

Female Madness in the Popular Press

Historians of scientific publishing (Dawson et al. 2004, 2020; Cantor and Shuttleworth 2004) have shown that popular science (science for and by the public) made up a significant portion of the content of a variety of periodicals published during the nineteenth century. Science and medicine were an integral part of the popular periodical press in this period, 'appearing not only in avowedly scientific articles, but also in other forms of narrative including fictional representations, glancing asides in political reports, and caricatures and allusions in comic magazines' (Dawson et al. 2004, p. 1). Plenty of medical content was published in periodicals not marketed as scientific, for example in literary magazines. This content was intended for lay consumption and was a recognition of public interest in medical and scientific topics. As Megan Coyer (2017) has shown in her study of Edinburgh's literary periodicals, medical content for a popular audience ranged from articles written by specialists to fictionalised accounts of medical practice for entertainment purposes.

The proliferation of scientific content outside of professional journals meant that readers were well-versed in current developments in many areas of science and medicine. The marketability of this content was such that many titles were published with the sole purpose of communicating scientific information to a non-specialist readership. As Bernard Lightman has argued, the 'transformation of nineteenth-century publishing opened up opportunities for making science more accessible to a new polity of middle and working-class readers' (Lightman 2016, p. 346). The wide availability and diversity of periodicals meant that the general public could keep abreast of the latest findings and join in by publishing their own research, facilitating the creation of non-specialist or amateur groups who actively participated in scientific discussions and endeavours.

The theory and treatment of insanity was just one of a plethora of topics related to the medical sciences which captured readerly interest. In the decades following the passage of the 1845 Lunacy Act, articles and features about mental disease regularly appeared in publications intended for a broader audience. There were inevitable differences in content and style between articles produced for scientific publications and those written for a non-medical readership, and articles published in general periodicals during this period tend to be lightly informative and accessible to a broad readership (Peterson 1994; Cooter and Pumphrey 1994; Cantor and Shuttleworth 2004; Shuttleworth and Charnley 2016).

However, the presence of theories of madness in the popular press shows that at least a certain amount of psychiatric knowledge had entered colloquial discourse. The fact that lay audiences would want to read about psychiatric medicine was not controversial. From essays on the brain, to passing references to hysteria in news articles, audiences were expected to be familiar with mental disease, and to be interested in reading about it and discussing it.

Content on the female mind was part of this trend. For example, *Reynold's Miscellany* ran a piece in their regular column 'Our Medical Corner,' entitled 'On Some Affections Incidental to Women—Hysteria' (1855). *Reynold's* was a cheap weekly, featuring different kinds of amusing or instructive content such as serialised fiction and informational articles. 'Our Medical Corner' was a column dedicated to educating readers on the fundamentals of various diseases. In this particular issue, a Dr Tilt (likely a tongue-in-cheek pseudonym) described the nature and symptoms of hysteria and offered guidance on the prevention of the disease in young women. This kind of light-touch, friendly medical advice fitted well with *Reynold's* house style and entertaining yet informative content. Helpful articles written by doctors were common across the general periodical press and contributions by general practitioners on female insanity should be understood within this context.

Later in the century, the discussion of mental disease within the popular press became more rigorous, covering both physiology and clinical presentation in more detail. This mirrored the increasing use of scientific methodologies within medicine at the time, as the profession became more focused on the pathology of disease. The distinguished Harley Street physician Alfred T. Schofield kept up a regular contribution to the weekly penny paper *Leisure Hour* during the 1880s and 90s, covering various health issues including nervous disease in both women and men. Schofield was interested in psychology and later went on to publish treatises on the role of the unconscious mind, functional nervous disease, and the treatment of nervous disorders through mental therapeutics (psychological therapies) (Schofield 1899, 1904, 1905). His column was a serious attempt to communicate scientific information to the lay reader, intended to educate through the careful explanation of detailed medical topics such as 'Nervousness and Hysteria' (Schofield 1889), 'Inside a Brain' (Schofield 1888a), and 'A Bad Headache' (Schofield 1888b).

Though intended to inform, medical content aimed at the layman did not always contain the most accurate information. I.P. Davis, MD, wrote an article entitled 'Hygiene for Girls', published in the October 1883 number of the moralistic miscellany *Golden Hours: A Monthly Magazine for Family and General Reading*. Priced at sixpence, the monthly was an affordable illustrated periodical with a foundation in Christian values. Davis's essay is clearly influenced by these values. The essay is a didactic piece, intended to teach readers the basics of nervous physiology and how to prevent disease in young girls. Davis describes how the term '"sympathy", when used in a physiological sense, means the influence through which action or irritation of one organ produces a corresponding action or irritation of another organ more or less remote' (Davis 1883, p. 593). He goes on to say that hysteria is a sympathetic affection, 'very much more common among women than among men' and 'in many cases its cause exists in some disease or irritation of some organ particular to women, particularly the womb' (Davis 1883, p. 593). Such theories were an outdated explanation of nerve action by the 1880s, when Jean-Martin Charcot's theories of hysteria as resulting from nervous weakness and degeneration were more current. To make matters worse, Davis then abandons science entirely and blames the prevalence of hysteria in modern society on young girls reading 'poisonous fiction' about 'spirit-mediums,' 'animated manikins,' 'detectives' and 'Indian fighters' (Davis 1883, p. 596). Reading fiction had little to do with contemporary theories of nervous disorder. These comments appear to be Davis's personal views about an activity he considered unsuitable for young girls, views which may well have been shared by the conservative Christian readership of *Golden Hours*. Indeed, it does not seem that Davis was particularly qualified to write about mental disease.

None of the three authors mentioned here were specialists in psychiatry, although Schofield was interested in the brain. Significantly, the discussion of female madness in the nineteenth-century periodical press does not appear to have been undertaken by mind doctors themselves. Although sometimes signed by an MD like Schofield or Davis, most contributions on female madness are unattributed or written by a staff journalist. Although the custom of anonymous journalism prevalent throughout the nineteenth century means that it is difficult to know for certain who was authoring such pieces, it is notable that psychiatric knowledge was not being visibly communicated by experts in the field. Such authorship was crucial to the way in which information about the female mind and its diseases was consumed by non-specialist audiences, not least because of the issues of accuracy seen in the example above. Yet mind doctors well known for their textbooks and other scientific publications apparently shunned equal prominence in the popular press.

Of the thirteen authors of psychiatric textbooks discussed in the previous chapter, only a handful produced signed articles for the general press, and typically only one or two throughout their lifetime.[2] Most of the essays written by these mind doctors were in relation to the practical and social aspects of their discipline, such as those particulars relating to lunacy law and medical jurisprudence, or changes to asylum management. George Fielding Blandford, for example, authored an essay on the issue of criminal responsibility, entitled 'Acquitted on the Grounds of Insanity' and published in the *Cornhill Magazine* (Fielding Blandford 1865). Likewise, Daniel Hack Tuke published two essays for *Macmillan's Magazine*, both dealing with concerns of the day: 'Modern Life and Insanity' (Hack Tuke 1877), and 'Broadmoor, and our Criminal Lunatics' (Hack Tuke 1878). Forbes Benignus Winslow also made many contributions to discussions on criminal law during the latter decades of the century, not only with published essays, but by responding to debate in the correspondence sections of several periodicals. Changes to lunacy law from 1845 onwards were important developments for both the profession and the public as the nation worried about certification, wrongful confinement, and rising asylum populations. It therefore stands to reason that mind doctors felt they had something to offer on this topic; it was one which would fundamentally impact their developing field.

Nevertheless, the relative invisibility of textbook authors in the periodical press, particularly in comparison to the sheer volume of articles on the subject of insanity, is striking. The lack of attribution to mind doctors does not necessarily mean that they did not write for non-specialist publications, either anonymously or under a pseudonym. As Dawson et al. (2004) have demonstrated, scientific articles frequently appeared in the higher brow general periodicals and were clearly authored by people with an advanced level of disciplinary knowledge. The new monthly reviews of the 1860s, for example, 'emulated the intellectual debates taking place in

[2] These results were obtained through full-name searches for textbook authors over five main periodical indexes/databases: ProQuest British Periodicals, Gale Nineteenth-Century Periodicals, ProQuest C19, the Waterloo Directory, and the Curran Index. Searches were limited to 1845–95, as well as 'author' and 'article' fields.

societies, clubs, and conversaziones' (Dawson et al. 2004, p. 20). If mind doctors did publish unsigned articles in these journals such anonymity may have simply been custom, though it could be an indication of deeper concerns surrounding professional propriety, as discretion was a major worry in a field dealing with such a sensitive issue as mental illness. It is difficult to know for certain but there are several factors which were likely influential in mind doctors' choosing not to publish in non-specialist journals (or at least not to publish under their own name).

For a nineteenth-century mind doctor to publish a scientific work in the general periodical press, there needed to be a specific benefit in doing so as this activity would not have been a customary part of their daily working lives. One benefit was payment for articles published. The fact that few articles have been identified as written by professionals indicates that there was a lack of opportunity in this regard. This is supported by what we already know about nineteenth-century psychiatry: for most early alienists, their living was made through asylum work and, towards the end of the century, hospital appointments, rather than publications (Scull 1979, 1993). Another benefit to writing for the periodical press was the enhancement of professional reputation for the author. Publishing scientific findings across the specialist press was an established method of increasing professional standing by the mid-nineteenth century, across disciplines (Csiszar 2018). From the 1870s, signed authorship prevailed in the press as a whole and, according to Dawson et al., 'professional scientific writers were able to establish distinct authorial personas' in the non-specialist press as well, exhibiting their 'expertise and credibility on particular topics' through 'expressing consistent individual opinions across a range of different articles' (Dawson et al. 2004, p. 21). Mind doctors do not appear to have taken advantage of these opportunities. Although many textbook authors were active contributors to medical journals and wrote other long form works such as treatises on insanity, they remained absent or invisible in the public realm.

This suggests that writing for the non-medical press was simply not useful to them as a method of career progression. Psychiatry was a developing and relatively close-knit discipline throughout the nineteenth century. Due to the stigma which still surrounded mental illness and its doctors, it was not a particularly public-facing profession. Although there was strong public interest in madness, mind doctors themselves tended to be heavily focused on their asylum roles and related communities, such as the Medico-Psychological Association. A publication record of textbooks and treatises was therefore sufficient to establish professional reputation for those who worked in the field. This was unlike other medical specialties during this period (Brown 2011; Moulds 2021). Rick Rylance has shown that nineteenth-century mind doctors 'lacked an established disciplinary identity, career structure, and specialist outlets for publication'; the profession was 'eclectic in its sources, dispersed in personnel, and generalist in orientation' (Rylance 2004, p. 239–41). In short, Victorian psychiatry was 'the *making* of a discipline' (Rylance 2004, p. 241). The specific process of discipline formation which occurred within the mind sciences was thus likely a major cause of the absence of professional authorship in the lay press.

The impact of this was a lack of public visibility of psychiatric expertise, meaning that the public had no clear source of authority for information on the mind. The plethora of content on female insanity in the general periodical press, from gossip to more serious essays, was a product of this absence of expertise and undoubtedly contributed to the slippage between cultural and scientific belief about women's madness. There was, however, one mind doctor who *did* publish in the non-specialist press, and under his own signature: Henry Maudsley. This chapter will now explore why Maudsley might have been inclined to produce an essay for a general audience, a readership his colleagues avoided.

Henry Maudsley and the Publication of 'Sex in Mind and in Education'

Henry Maudsley was one of the leading alienists of the Victorian period, forging his career just as the profession was becoming established as a respected field of medicine. Working at Wakefield, Brentwood, and Manchester Royal Asylums during his early career, he gained a number of respected positions at London hospitals in the 1860s alongside the proprietorship of a lucrative private asylum, The Lawn. He obtained membership of the Medico-Psychological Association (MPA) in 1858 and the coveted position of co-editor of the organisation's *Journal of Mental Science* in 1863. During this time, Maudsley also published several well received articles in scientific journals, as well as two treatises: *The Physiology and Pathology of Mind* (1867), and *Body and Mind: An Inquiry into their Mutual Connection and Influence* (1871) (Turner 2010). However, it was not until 1874 that Maudsley wrote for the popular periodical press.

This turn towards a non-specialist audience had its catalyst in the career difficulties he had begun to face in the early 1870s.

Despite his excellent publication record and commendable professional advancements, Maudsley was not well liked within the mind doctoring community and was considered by colleagues to hold somewhat controversial opinions. His work was dominated by a belief in the hereditary and degenerative nature of mental illness, which he came to view as largely incurable once the patient exhibited signs of disease. Although he was well acquainted with the latest research, and his adherence to evolutionary psychiatry was not at odds with late-Victorian medicine, his pessimism isolated him from many of his fellow alienists (Showalter 1987). Relations became strained between himself and other MPA members and the tension came to a head when Maudsley's 1871 MPA Presidential Address mocked several important colleagues, including Thomas Smith Clouston, and offended the profession as a whole—bad blood from which he never quite recovered (Maudsley 1871a; Turner 1988; Scull et al. 1996).

On a personal level, Maudsley was felt by his contemporaries to be abrasive and difficult; Clouston in particular thought him to be a sceptic and a doomsayer. George Henry Savage wrote Maudsley's obituary for the *Journal of Mental Science* in 1918 and barely hid his dislike behind duty-bound politeness. Although he granted that Maudsley was a 'close critic and a careful student of current medical knowledge,' Savage could not help remarking that his subject was 'not a clubbable man' (Savage 1918, pp. 118–119). Maudsley was someone 'who seemed to prefer solitude,' and was 'uncompromising' in his beliefs (Savage 1918, p. 117). It appears that he had no qualms about openly criticising those who fell short of these standards, as Savage noted from his own experience: 'I have a collection, which I have headed "Maudsley's Fire." I shall never forget some of these, in which he criticised either something I had written, or some opinion I had given' (Savage 1918, p. 118). Maudsley's 'very strong feelings' on the treatment of the insane seemed to be at the root of many of these missives, Savage receiving some 'rather sarcastic communications from him in reference to forcible feeding' (Savage 1918, p. 119). For his contemporaries, Maudsley was an inconvenient person, both for his scientific views and his personal qualities. Savage's obituary paints a picture of a man who was uncomfortable in his professional community and who often felt as if 'the way things were done' was against his vision of how they should be.

Given his professional circumstances, it is unsurprising that Maudsley may have wanted to advance his prospects. By the 1870s, he was also dissatisfied with life at the head of an asylum, possibly because of his beliefs about the incurability of asylum patients. He began to divest himself of his ownership of The Lawn in 1874. Andrew Scull et al. (1996) have argued convincingly that it was at this point that Maudsley began manoeuvring to establish himself outside of the narrow alienist community. He planned to do so by being one of the first psychiatrists to set up a private clinic, catering to what he hoped would be the lucrative clientele of the health-conscious upper classes, prone to nervous disorders. This was an unusual career path. Only a few of the most prominent physicians had ever consulted on insanity outside of a state or private asylum—most notably John Munro, who had advised elite patients (including the doctors of King George III) in the previous century (Macintyre and Munro 2015). It was therefore a bold career move and to successfully execute it Maudsley needed to boost his reputation amongst the wider medical community and lay elite. A well-placed journal article, on a subject of importance, would reach the desired audiences and hopefully bolster his personal and professional image. In April 1874, Maudsley succeeded in securing just such an article, when the *Fortnightly Review* published his 'Sex in Mind and in Education' (Maudsley 1874).

In the essay, he responded to American physician Edward Clarke's (1873) recently published book, *Sex in Education; or, a Fair Chance for the Girls*. Focusing on the perils of co-education, which was then causing controversy in the United States, Clarke described what he perceived as the risks of this policy to the health of both women and the nation. Clarke believed that co-education (the practice of educating boys and girls together, in the same way) was wearing girls out to such a degree that it made them liable to nervous ill-health and reproductive problems later in life. In writing his response, Maudsley's purpose was to bring these issues to bear on the education of British women and demonstrate how the mind sciences might provide evidence of such grave dangers. According to Maudsley and Clarke, the physiology of the female mind prevented women from competing with men in the intellectual sphere.

'Sex in Mind and in Education' was Maudsley's first article to appear outside of the specialist press. Opportunely timed at the point of his withdrawal from asylum doctoring, it was calculated to engage the public's attention and ease his transition into private practice by showcasing his medical views in the best possible light. Female education, the hot topic of the moment, was the ideal choice of subject matter as it gave Maudsley maximum exposure. The movement for reform in female education had been steadily gaining momentum during the preceding decades (Rowold 1996, 2011). In 1849, Elizabeth Jesser Reid had pioneered higher education for women by opening Bedford College in London, with the intention of providing a non-sectarian curriculum. More opportunities arose for women from the mid-1860s. Cambridge and Oxford offered local examinations to girls. In June 1868 the University of London established the General Examination for Women for female students, enabling them to gain a Certificate of Proficiency. More women had also begun to open their own institutions, specifically for female students: in Cambridge Emily Davies established the first women's college in 1869 (which became Girton), and Henry Sedgwick and Anna Jemima Clough formed Newnham College soon after. Provincial universities were also receiving their charters at this time, and the federal Victoria University (out of which Manchester and Liverpool Universities would form) admitted women on equal terms from 1880.

Women's rights were discussed across the board as campaigners pushed for female emancipation in all areas, from the home to workplace. In 1857 the Matrimonial Causes Act had made it possible for a woman to obtain a divorce from her husband, yet the Contagious Disease Acts of the 1860s controversially legalised forced medical inspection of women suspected of prostitution, though the law was later repealed. These changes engendered much fierce debate between those who supported and those who opposed reform. The discursive space in which 'Sex in Mind and in Education' appeared was one in which the nature and role of women's bodies was seen as fundamental to society. Katharina Rowold (1996) has argued that 'Sex in Mind and in Education' went to the core of these debates. Maudsley's essay answered questions that were gripping the nation: 'Was the mind sexed? If so, what were the mental characteristics and abilities of women? […] What was the relationship between the female mind and the body? And what were the implications of knowing the answers to such questions for the opening up of higher education to women?' (Rowold 1996, p. 1). The 'model of the "reproductive body"' was crucial to these discussions, which were joined not only by Maudsley but by numerous other physicians weighing the issue throughout the 1870s (Rowold 1996, p. 8). Maudsley was thus wading in on a popular subject and his point of view surely proved satisfactory to many readers less inclined to reform.

Maudsley's article was also timed to respond directly to advances in female higher education which were underway as he wrote the piece and as it went to press. These included successes in the campaign for women's access to medical education (Elston 1986; Thompson 1998; Crowther and Dupree 2007; McIntyre 2014). Elizabeth Garrett Anderson, the first female doctor to qualify in Britain, had opened the New Hospital for Women in 1872 and was actively campaigning for women to be admitted to medical degrees whilst proving that women could work in the field through leading by example. Likewise, in the early months of 1874, Sophia Jex-Blake, one of the leading figures of the fight for women's access to medical education, founded the London School of Medicine for Women. Jex-Blake was one of thirty-nine women to attend classes in medicine at the University of Edinburgh, the first British medical school to accept female students in any capacity. Although Jex-Blake matriculated in medicine in 1869, the university made it more and more difficult for her and the other women students to attend classes and ultimately rejected them from the degree programme in 1873. However, their experience marked a turning point in women's entry into medicine, leading to Jex-Blake striking out on her own in the English capital.

This posed a threat to the male dominated profession and was doubtless a topic which Maudsley felt strongly about, but it was also one which would have interested those general practitioners with wealthy client bases whom he was trying to attract. Worryingly, there was also talk of the University of London admitting women to its degree examinations and the board passed a vote in favour less than a week after the publication of the *Fortnightly* April number (Orme 1874). This was a crucial development for the women's movement and Maudsley's article could not have come at a more opportune time for the generation of publicity.

The choice of the *Fortnightly Review* for publication was a strategic one. An elite monthly publishing serial fiction and topical reviews, the *Fortnightly* was founded in 1865 for a new middle-class reading market. It was priced at half a crown, which narrowed its audience to a well-to-do community of readers—just the kind of individuals who could pay for the private consultations Maudsley was hoping to offer. Then edited by John Morley, the *Fortnightly* had an intellectual reputation and often published serious essays on contemporary political or scientific topics (Turner 2009). The periodical was thus a well-known and respected organ which gave a platform of legitimacy and respectability to Maudsley's views. Despite this, there were other likely places for

Maudsley to publish his article, such as the *Westminster Review*, which had a long-standing reputation for producing scientific content and had published work from such famous names as Herbert Spencer and T. H. Huxley. However, the *Fortnightly*'s monthly schedule made for more up-to-the-minute content than the quarterly *Westminster*, which by the 1870s appeared quite old fashioned.[3] Crucially, the *Fortnightly* also had a policy of attributed authorship (Turner 2000; Small 2003; Nash 2010). In publishing a signed article, Maudsley ensured that he would receive recognition amongst lay readers, who might be reminded of his reputation as a scientific writer when choosing a doctor to treat their nervous ills. It is also worth noting that the *Fortnightly* also always advertised its leaders in the week prior to the release of a new number, potentially generating opportunity for further exposure for Maudsley.

Maudsley's article was a rare example within nineteenth-century psychiatry of publicly visible authorship. In 'Sex in Mind and in Education', Maudsley spoke with authority to an audience outside of the profession and, crucially, spoke with the assumption that such a readership would be interested in what he had to say. Weighing in on the popular debate on female emancipation, Maudsley's contribution attracted attention as he took the unusual step of using medical evidence to answer a social question. Maudsley's motivation in writing the article is crucial to how such theories came to be used in this way. The publication of his essay in the general periodical press had much to do with Maudsley's exceptional personality, which led him to seek work outside of the asylum in private practice. Unlike his fellow alienists, Maudsley had a reason to publish in the non-specialist press. His desire for his work to be seen, hence its publication in a non-medical journal, and his choice of subject matter, caused him to place his ideas on the female mind in a context altogether different from that of a textbook or treatise, shifting them to a social and cultural register only latent in his medical texts.

This presents a unique opportunity to understand the reciprocal relationship between social ideology and gendered psychiatric theory in the late nineteenth century. In 'Sex in Mind and in Education', Maudsley used clinical knowledge to justify the position of women within Victorian society, specifically their domestic role as wives and mothers and the

[3] The periodical's name belied its publication schedule. Although it was published every two weeks in its first year, thereafter the *Fortnightly Review* appeared monthly and fell firmly in the camp of the new monthly magazines.

consequent limitations imposed upon their education. A close reading of the essay can therefore reveal how the gendered ideologies which informed the creation of psychiatric theories about women were in turn reinforced through the manipulation of these very theories in support of a social agenda.

Maudsley's Article and the Social Application of Gendered Psychiatric Theory

In 'Sex in Mind and in Education', Maudsley argued that girls should not be educated in the same manner as boys, and by extension, that women should not be allowed to participate in higher education in the same way as men. This argument was grounded in his belief that 'there are significant differences between the sexes,' differences which were fundamental to the 'organisation' of the species (Maudsley 1874, p. 466). According to Maudsley, the biological disparity between men and women was insurmountable; 'come what may in the assimilation of female and male education and labour [...] it will not be possible to transform a woman into a man' (Maudsley 1874, p. 466). The differentiation between sexes, Maudsley believed, was due to a woman's 'special functions,' which in turn determined her 'special sphere of development and activity' in society (Maudsley 1874, p. 466). In other words, to her reproductive capacities which fitted her for her domestic role as wife and mother. These special functions were so important to a woman's health, that to ignore them would result in disaster. Thus, although women might be able to compete on an intellectual level with men, Maudsley argued that they could not do so 'without serious injury' to 'health and strength' (Maudsley 1874, p. 466).

Maudsley's reasoning was rooted in Laycock's theory of reflex action between the organs and nerves, and furthermore, to a belief in the role of the female reproductive organs in maintaining or disrupting the balance of mental health in women. The 'energy of a human body being a definite and not inexhaustible quality,' and the female reproductive organs requiring such a large amount of that energy, Maudsley and other mind doctors believed that there was 'nothing more necessary to the preservation of female health' than the complete regularity of such organs being sustained (Maudsley 1874, p. 467). As we have seen, mind doctors unanimously agreed that influence was felt between the female mind and reproductive body. Maudsley's own medical works demonstrate his support of these theories. In his 1870 treatise, *Body and Mind*, he argued that there existed 'the closest physiological consent between the different organs,' in consequence of which 'the derangement of an internal organ, acting upon the brain, may engender, by pathological sympathy, morbid feelings and related ideas' (Maudsley 1871b, p. 81). In women, the action of the reproductive organs was particularly important in producing 'special bodily and mental characters' that shaped the nature and function of the female brain (Maudsley 1871b, p. 82). In particular, Maudsley argued, 'the monthly activity of the ovaries'—or menstruation—'has a notable effect on the mind and body' and may become 'an important cause of mental derangement' (Maudsley 1871b, p. 87). Even without succumbing to outright insanity, he wrote, 'most women at that time are susceptible, irritable, and capricious' (Maudsley 1871b, p. 87).

The ideas which Maudsley outlined in 'Sex in Mind and in Education' were therefore consistent with the psychiatric theories he supported in his earlier works for a specialist audience. There was one important difference, however, between the *Fortnightly* article and Maudsley's medical treatises: the application of such theories outside of the clinical realm. In *Body and Mind*, Maudsley was writing for an audience of medical professionals. Like psychiatric textbooks, these treatises were intended to be read by a community of mind doctors and other medical practitioners and Maudsley wrote only of the relationship between women's health and insanity. Whilst introducing his first major publication, *The Physiology and Pathology of Mind*, Maudsley had written: 'the aim which I have had in view throughout this work has been [...] to treat of mental phenomena from a physiological [...] point of view' (Maudsley 1867a, p. vi). Outlining the physiology of the female body and its impact upon the mind, Maudsley described the reciprocal action of nerve processes, how this might result in insanity, and what the symptoms of mental disease might be. Catering for a specialist audience, he was interested in demonstrating his expertise and putting forward a scientific thesis; any consideration of socio-cultural issues would have been distinctly out of place in such a work.

However, in his *Fortnightly* essay, Maudsley was writing for a diverse readership of the educated middle and upper-middle classes, in a publication concerned with the political and social issues of the day. Furthermore, he was intending to capture the attention of a lay public who might potentially form a lucrative client base for his future private practice. Simply regurgitating the dry theories espoused in his treatises would not be sufficient. Maudsley needed to demonstrate the importance of psychiatry as a discipline and position himself as a top doctor in the field, one who understood the role his specialism could play in questions of national importance. Unlike in his earlier writing, Maudsley was concerned to highlight the social as well as medical pertinence of his theories. In particular, he needed to illustrate how psychiatric evidence of the gendered mind validated an educational system based on sex difference.

Maudsley's essay draws on these theories of conservation of energy for evidence against the inclusion of girls and women in higher education. He insists that nothing is more important than that menstruation should take place 'regularly and completely' (Maudsley 1874, p. 467). For this to occur, women must take care to allow enough bodily energy to be reserved for the performance of their monthly cycle, by avoiding 'an excessive mental drain as well as the natural physical drain which is so great at that time' (Maudsley 1874, p. 467). If they failed to do so, 'irregularity, imperfection, arrest, or excess' could occur during menstruation, and 'pallor, lassitude, debility, sleeplessness, headache, neuralgia, and then worse ills' would follow in consequence (Maudsley 1874, p. 474). This prescription was problematic for aspiring girls, considering the amount of brain power which might be needed for academic success. The advent of menstruation at puberty was an especially critical period, being one in which girls underwent bodily changes whilst they were likely to be in school (Shail 2010). Maudsley notes rather condescendingly that the fact 'the development of puberty does draw heavily upon the vital resources of the female constitution, needs not to be pointed out to those who know the nature of the important physiological changes which then take place' (Maudsley 1874, p. 467).

Crucially, menstruation was but one of the challenges jeopardising women's access to a full education, a symptom of the fundamental difference in character between the female and male body and thus the female and male mind. As Maudsley emphatically put it, 'they cannot choose but to be women; cannot rebel successfully against the tyranny of their organisation, the complete development and function whereof must take place after its kind. [...] It is the plain statement of a physiological fact' (Maudsley 1874, p. 468). Although 'it is not that girls have not ambition, nor that they fail generally to run the intellectual race which is set before them,' it is that intellectual overwork will cause 'lifelong suffering' brought on by disregard for the 'greater instability' of female nerve-centres (Maudsley 1874, p. 473). He rails against the schools which, through co-education, catalyse a rash of nervous breakdowns that might have been 'predicted on physiological grounds' (Maudsley 1874, p. 473).

Maudsley thus establishes causality between a social issue (co-education) and a pathology (mental disease in female pupils), a theory he believed to be substantiated by psychiatric evidence of the weaker female brain. It is clear from 'Sex in Mind and in Education' that, in Maudsley's view, psychiatry provided scientific support for the ideology of separate spheres (of which single-sex education was merely one facet) by revealing the physiology which necessitated the social system. Yet, medical theories on the female mind were formed using the very same gendered ideologies which Maudsley is here using such theory to reinforce. The use of psychiatry as evidence in support of a social policy exposes how Maudsley's beliefs, and those of his profession, were intertwined with the ideological biases of Victorian culture.

Arguing that the influence of women's reproductive function 'pervades and affects essentially their entire beings,' Maudsley suggests that 'proper regard to the physical nature of women means attention given, in their training [...] to their foreordained work as mothers and nurses of children' (Maudsley 1874, p. 471). Women, the article states, are 'manifestly endowed with qualities of mind which specially fit them to stimulate and foster the first growths of intelligence in children,' with 'intimate and special sympathies' particular to mothers (Maudsley 1874, p. 472). Likewise, 'the female qualities of mind which correlate her sexual character adapt her, as her sex does, to be the helpmate and companion of man' (Maudsley 1874, p. 472). Educating her for 'these important offices' should cause no mental harm, whereas 'laborious days of intellectual exercise' would only be a miserable and ultimately failed resistance against her essential nature (Maudsley 1874, p. 471). Female education should correlate with women's biological destiny. Maudsley argues that the disastrous effects of co-education merely 'show that the main reason of woman's position lies in her nature' (Maudsley 1874, p. 478).

Such claims fostered the Victorian ideal of the 'angel in the house', the primacy and sanctity of motherhood, and the domestic and submissive role of women in marriage. These ideals were naturalised within psychiatry through gendered theories of mental disease focused on the reproductive organs. The importance of the domestic ideal to Victorian society generated a strongly held belief in the significance of reproduction for the female body; this belief then shaped psychiatric theories about the female mind. The cause-and-effect which Maudsley outlines in the article is therefore manifestly circular logic. Women's unfitness for education outside of the domestic sphere is justified by claims about the fragility of the female mind due to the impact of the reproductive system; a theory which was itself the product of a biological essentialism that aligned motherhood with the essence of what it means to be a woman. Such arguments reveal how gendered psychiatric theory, shaped by the ideology of separate spheres, is in turn used by Maudsley to support the confinement of women to the home and refuse them the same educational opportunities as men.

For Maudsley, this biological essentialism was validated by his staunch belief in evolutionary theory. The evolutionary development of humankind had irreversibly formed women into maternal creatures. In his 1867 article for the *Journal of Mental Science*, 'On Some of the Causes of Insanity', Maudsley had outlined his views on the topic. He stressed the 'stupendous progress of the human race' through time, in which the 'fierce struggle for existence' had shaped the sexual roles of men and women (Maudsley 1867b, pp. 490–491). This fight for survival, over the centuries, had resulted in 'the appropriation by man, the stronger sex, of all the means of subsistence by labour, to almost the entire exclusion of women' (Maudsley 1867b, p. 491). However, because 'women are indispensable to the comfort of men's lives,' they have not been 'crushed out of existence' but 'kept in a state of subjection and dependence, and in such state protected' (Maudsley 1867b, p. 491). Maudsley believed that the ministering role of women under this system had ensured that 'through generations her character has been formed with that chief aim' of serving men. Consequently, the sexual life of women had been 'undesignedly developed at the expense of the intellectual' (Maudsley 1867a, pp. 231–232).

In the *Fortnightly*, Maudsley asks, 'does it not appear that in order to assimilate the female to the male mind it would be necessary to undo the life-history of mankind from its earliest commencement?' (Maudsley 1874, p. 471). Woman's position as a companion to man and her child bearing capacity 'must always have rendered, and must continue to render, most of her activity domestic' (Maudsley 1874, p. 478). He refutes the feminist argument that, historically, women have 'been in the position of a slave kept in forcible subjection by the superior physical force of men,' assuring the reader that 'she has been a slave content with her bondage' (Maudsley 1874, p. 478). According to Maudsley, the true woman 'does not care to be free,' only desiring to fulfil the noble calling of her maternal nature (Maudsley 1874, p. 478). It is because the female body is physically weaker and essentially fitted for reproduction that women have been placed in such bondage, and thus it is natural that they should not wish to rebel against it. Here again we see evidence of Maudsley's circular arguments, as evolutionary theory is used to justify the domestic role of women, at the same time as their domestic role provides evidence for such a hypothesis.

Maudsley's prejudices are revealed when the article turns to the long-term consequences of female education and the havoc it will cause for society. In principle and in practice, co-education represented an attempt to throw off millions of years of evolution and reform womanhood into a new, semi-masculine type. Maudsley argues that the mental disease already present in schoolgirls is but a precursor of the great ills to come, the first sign of degeneration caused by an attempt to fly in the face of nature. Co-education triggered nervous disease through reciprocal action between the brain and reproductive organs, making women barren or at least 'unfit for the best discharge of maternal functions' (Maudsley 1874, p. 475). Indeed, Maudsley predicts a society in which women would be unable to bear children, or only able to bear weak, degenerate types: 'it would be an ill thing [...] that we got the advantages of a quantity of female intellectual work at the price of a puny, enfeebled, and sickly race' (Maudsley 1874, p. 472). Motherhood is 'recklessly sacrificed in the acquirement of learning,' and 'in mind, as in body, the individual fails to reach the ideal of a complete and perfect womanhood' (Maudsley 1874, pp. 475–477). These well-educated yet incomplete women are 'a monstrosity- something which having ceased to be woman is yet not man' (Maudsley 1874, p. 477).

Maudsley's disgust is palpable in these lines, demonstrating just how integral reproductive function was to his conception of femininity. Without it, a woman could not be a woman, instead becoming something abhorrent: a transgression against nature. For Maudsley, 'the aim of female education should manifestly be the perfect development, not of manhood but of womanhood,' an education which supported the normative sex roles that were the foundation of Victorian masculinity and femininity (Maudsley 1874, p. 481). Although his purpose in writing for the *Fortnightly* was to capture public attention and promote the relevance of psychiatry as a discipline, it is evident that Maudsley felt extremely strongly about the topic, and that his own belief system was influential in the claims he made about the female mind. Chastising the female supporters of co-education, Maudsley draws the essay to a close with a macabre premonition: 'if they are wrong, the error will avenge itself upon them and upon their children, if they should ever have any' (Maudsley 1874, p. 482). In true doomsaying fashion, he is confident that the inexorable tide of evolution will ensure that the mistakes of these non-women will quickly pass out of the human race.

Fortunately, 'Sex in Mind and in Education' had little impact upon the opening of higher education for women, the expansion of which continued into the twentieth century. It did, however, provoke a huge public response, not least from some of the very women who would be so instrumental in the successful campaign for women's educational rights. In the months following the article's publication, an extensive debate ranged across numerous and varied publications as many readers weighed in on Maudsley's article and women's right to education. Clearly, Maudsley achieved the publicity he set out to attain. Yet, in using his medical training to publicly criticise female education, he created a discursive space for the discussion of these psychiatric theories amongst the lay public. Unfortunately for Maudsley, this meant that he had inadvertently opened his expertise to criticism by those outside of the psychiatric profession. By allowing a wide variety of people to have their say in print, the popular periodical press facilitated a greater range of interpretations of women's mental abilities, calling Maudsley's claims into doubt.

The Female Mind in Debate

In the early weeks of April 1874, Maudsley's article was picked up by a number of reviews (with a response in the *Saturday Review*, the *Westminster Review*, and the *Fortnightly* itself), a literary magazine (*Blackwood's Edinburgh Magazine*), and an intellectual weekly (the *Examiner*). These respondents came from diverse backgrounds, demonstrating just how central the issue of female education was to current affairs. Writers included both lay men and women, alongside female medical professionals, and their replies took a range of different forms as correspondence, opinion pieces or essays. The volume and variety of responses in the press also meant that, for perhaps the first time, psychiatric theories were widely discussed in a public forum between medical professionals and lay people. Following this debate allows us to understand how Maudsley's ideas were received and challenged across different readerships.

As the replies to his essay unfolded in the press, control over psychiatric knowledge moved away from Maudsley to these respondents, shifting from a single source of professional expertise to a diffuse, multitudinous, and conflicting group of voices. Medical theories about the female mind were reiterated, questioned or outright rejected in each contribution to the debate as writers competed for the authority to speak on the subject. The authorship of each response was thus integral to how ideas about the female mind were discussed, as each individual writer brought their own belief system to bear on the topic. In addition, the form of contribution and the specific publication each appeared in were instrumental to the shape these theories took at various moments. Textual form was therefore a key factor in the redevelopment of psychiatric theories outside of the professional realm, as the non-specialist press not only facilitated a greater range of interpretations of female madness, but actively shaped these articulations through the regulating power of genre and market audience.

Women's Voices

Significantly, the publication of 'Sex in Mind and in Education' in the non-specialist *Fortnightly Review* allowed for a much broader readership and audience engagement than that of nineteenth-century medical journals. This wider market was vital in provoking controversial debate as it enabled women to comment on medical theories about their own minds. This was a novel opportunity, even for women who were medically trained, as medical journals were male dominated forms of communication during this period. These periodicals were the publications of learned societies and institutions, which restricted membership to male medical professionals until late in the nineteenth century. Only members of the society could have their articles published in its journal (though anyone could read them). The British Medical Association, for example, produced and edited the *British Medical Journal* from 1840 and only opened membership to female doctors in 1892 (Elston 1986).[4] Individuals who were not medically qualified, male or female, were also unable to contribute to these publications (Brake 2000; Turner 2019). In popular

[4] The exception was Elizabeth Garrett Anderson who, having succeeded in qualifying as a doctor, had joined the Association through a legal loophole in 1873. She remained the only woman member for 19 years.

discussions of Maudsley's essay, female writers were therefore able to demonstrate publicly, for perhaps the first time, why they should have the right to be heard, staking a claim to authority by virtue of their sex as they capitalised on the idea that women might know more about their own bodies than any male doctor. The first flurry of responses to appear in the press were all from female correspondents, eager to have their say.

The first periodical to publish a reply to Maudsley's article was the *Examiner*. The frequency of its publication schedule ensured that it was ahead of other periodicals in running the initial response to 'Sex in Mind and in Education.' Priced at three pence a number during the 1870s, it was a literary weekly with a radical outlook that was accessible to the middle classes (Bersohn 2009). The periodical's reformist tone meant that female emancipation in all its forms was a regular topic amongst its pages and comment on Maudsley's essay would have been just the thing to appeal to the *Examiner*'s readers. In fact, the first reply the periodical published was placed in its correspondence section. Entitled 'Sex in Education' and signed 'H.T.', the letter ran on April 18th, 1874, two weeks after Maudsley's article appeared in the *Fortnightly* (H.T. 1874). The *Examiner* regularly published readers' letters (some of them commissioned) and the correspondence section was a particularly important feature of the publication, appearing prominently near the middle and taking up around a fifth of each number. As a weekly, the *Examiner* could engage with its readers through regular letters and thus create a unified and consistent identity for the publication and its audience.

Written from a prestigious address (Hyde Park Gardens) and taking a progressive and humorous tone in favour of co-education, H.T.'s letter is exactly suited to a higher-class periodical that prided itself on being concerned with intellectual affairs. Women's education was discussed across several numbers during this period and given how neatly the letter fits with the *Examiner*'s politics and personality, H.T. was likely a regular reader who identified with the periodical. The use of inclusive pronouns when talking about the issue of women's education, as well as the attitude of solidarity, also indicates that H.T. was a woman (not unusual for the weekly, which had a cross-gender readership). H.T. opens by lamenting the 'meddling interest' the medical profession had lately taken in women's 'health and occupations' (H.T. 1874, p. 399). She begins by 'question[ing] the taste which led Dr Maudsley to select a periodical of this nature for the publication of his views on [...] the physical organisation of women,' protesting against the impropriety of discussing such intimate medical details in a 'paper for general circulation' (H.T. 1874, p. 399).[5] Determined to avoid discussion of physiological details herself, she rejects medical authority outright, calling on female experience and common sense to provide a solution to the question of female education: 'There are mothers, daughters, and sisters amongst us who think they are quite capable of judging and finding out by accumulated experience what is good for their bodies and minds, under the ordinary circumstances of health, as any doctor' (H.T. 1874, p. 399).

This tongue-in-cheek tone is a key feature of H.T.'s style. She mocks Maudsley's bluster about the dissolution of sex, asking how merely educating women is 'to effect the miracle of changing them into men' and suggesting that perhaps it is the 'same metamorphosis as that which changes a man, who has propounded something foolish, into "an old woman"' (H.T. 1874, p. 399). Quoting Maudsley's argument that '"some have thought that a girl's passion for a doll evinces even at that time a fore-feeling of her future functions,"' H.T. laughingly remarks that it is 'within the experience of many mothers to have had daughters who detested dolls and sons who had a tender regard for them,' but that it had probably never occurred to them that 'differences in their children's tastes were "fore-feelings." [...] Only the prophetic soul of "some" could perceive this' (H.T. 1874, p. 400). By subverting Maudsley's arguments with hyperbolic language for comedic effect, H.T. undermines his authority to speak on the subject. She is also indirectly undercutting the male, medical jurisdiction over the female mind which Maudsley both embodies and symbolises. Humour is therefore central to H.T.'s dismissal of Maudsley's views and the rejection of his claims to expertise. Whilst this technique would have been out of place in a more serious essay, it fits perfectly with the discursive practices of a section of readers' letters. The greater scope for personal voice within the correspondence genre is integral to H.T.'s ability to utilise comedy in her writing, enabling her, as a (probably female) lay respondent, to challenge Maudsley by legitimising forms of debate other than theoretical reasoning.

[5] A full analysis of the issue of propriety in medical discussions in the non-specialist press is outside the scope of this chapter. However, it is worth noting that Maudsley's frank discussion of menstruation created a space where it was possible to talk about the intimate details of the female body, though not all those who responded to his article approved.

The *Examiner* published another reply to Maudsley's article two weeks later in the May 2nd number. Also titled 'Sex in Education', the response was written by Sophia Jex-Blake (1874), who, as we have seen, was a pioneering female physician and campaigner for women's right to medical education, having fought for her right to attend the University of Edinburgh medical school. She was thus a key figure in the debates on female higher education and had a vested interest in refuting Maudsley's claims. In March 1874, just before the publication of Maudsley's article, Jex-Blake had moved to London with the aim of opening the London School of Medicine for Women, which she succeeded in doing in October of that year. The *Examiner* had followed Jex-Blake's activities across several preceding numbers, and on May 2nd it also ran an article entitled 'Women and the Scottish Universities', which detailed her struggles and the Bill then in Parliament for the expansion of women's higher education (Bright 1874). The publication evidently shared the politics of Jex-Blake and her supporters and was a receptive periodical in which to place her response to Maudsley. As a non-specialist yet intellectual organ, the *Examiner* was an ideal place for women like Jex-Blake, who had medical training but were presently barred from the profession, to enter medical debates such as that on the female mind and education.

Rather than responding directly to Maudsley's article, which she admits she has never read, Jex-Blake uses its publicity as a platform to discuss female higher education in general. However, she is familiar with some of Maudsley's other works on female madness, including those in which he directly contradicts the *Fortnightly* article by ascribing 'a large proportion of insanity among women to the vapid and purposeless lives that so many of them are condemned to lead' (Jex-Blake 1874, p. 457). It is this inconsistency which she aims to expose in her letter, attacking a 'certain class of male writers [who] constantly assume that no labour is severe except that usually allocated to men, and that it is only when women venture to invade *that* field that they are likely to be overtasked' (Jex-Blake 1874, p. 457). She thus exposes the sexism inherent in these doctors' views and the 'delicious *naiveté*' which undermines their arguments (Jex-Blake 1874, p. 457). She even describes a Dr Henry Bennet who, after stressing that women should never undertake the kind of hard work required by the study of medicine, suggests that they would be ideally suited to employment in midwifery! However, even whilst Jex-Blake is concerned to highlight the misogynistic foundations of Maudsley's beliefs, she agrees that there are 'physiological laws' which 'can never be safely disregarded'

(Jex-Blake 1874, p. 457). Supporting his prescription that 'in girlhood *incessant* strain must always be a serious evil,' she argues that women need to remain aware of 'the dangers which they must avoid' (Jex-Blake 1874, p. 457). Nonetheless, she stresses that women's physiology has no adverse effects on their health or ability to work when properly managed, which she believes women are perfectly capable of doing without medical intervention. With a 'greater knowledge of physiology and hygiene,' women would be enabled to live 'full and useful lives' regardless of their reproductive capacities (Jex-Blake 1874, p. 457).

For Jex-Blake, these physiological laws may be facts of life, but there is no evidence that they pose a clinical concern. In revealing the inconsistencies and sexism behind Maudsley's theories on the female mind, she dismantles the connection between women's reproductive cycle and ill-health and incapacity. By undermining the medical arguments of Maudsley and his colleagues, both H.T. and Sophia Jex-Blake were refusing to acknowledge that female education held any danger at all to the health of women or the nation. The correspondence section of the *Examiner*, with its emphasis on rational discussion and openness to progressive viewpoints, enabled two very different women contributors to speak with authority on the issue of the female mind. Both draw their authority from their femaleness. By virtue of their own experiences as women, they claimed the right to reject or correct the views of the psychiatric profession. This was a claim that other, and equally different, female contributors would make before the debate was over.

It was in the number of the *Fortnightly* following Maudsley's article that the review published Elizabeth Garrett Anderson's (1874) essay 'Sex in Mind and Education: A Reply'. Garrett Anderson had written the response at the request of Frances Buss and Emily Davies, two women active in the campaign for female education who no doubt requested her help as Garrett Anderson was something of a figurehead for the movement (Burstyn 1980). Although the *Fortnightly* did not commission her article, it was likely keen to publish it. The review's nonpartisan policy allowed it to present diametrically opposed viewpoints across numbers to generate debate and, consequently, readership; the controversy between Maudsley and the poster-woman for female education was calculated to do just that. Garrett Anderson also benefited from the opportunity to respond to Maudsley within the same periodical, as it maximised her audience and gave her a high-profile platform from which to present her arguments. Her essay was, of course, in support of co-education, and the

Fortnightly was the perfect publication to relay her reformist ideals to a wide-reaching, intellectual readership.

Garrett Anderson was the first female doctor to qualify and register within Britain. In the years preceding the publication of 'Sex in Mind and in Education,' she took revolutionary steps towards forging a medical career. Obtaining an MD from the University of Paris in 1870, she was admitted to the British Medical Association in 1873—although the fact was not widely known until two years later. In 1871 she opened a hospital for women in Marylebone, employing only female medical staff, and had already established a private practice in which she treated women and children (Elston 2017). Garrett Anderson was thus a trailblazer not only in respect to the education of women, but also regarding women's access to the medical profession. Her article is significant as she was both a woman and a medically qualified contributor to the debate. Given the difficulties women faced in joining the medical profession, the staging of the debate in the general press gave her a unique opportunity to display her medical expertise.

Writing in the *Fortnightly*, Garrett Anderson was able to present her case to an influential and intellectual audience, separate from the medical establishment. This gave her the freedom to publicly challenge the received ideas of patriarchal mind doctors like Maudsley and position herself as a new kind of expert on women's health, undermining the monopoly of the all-male medical profession (Brock 2008). Crucially, Garrett Anderson's challenge to Maudsley rests not only on her professional training but on her sex too. Like Jex-Blake and H.T., she claims a greater right to speak on the topic of female health because of her womanhood. This claim had long been a key facet of Garrett Anderson's campaign for women's right to enter the medical professions; female doctors, she believed, would better understand female disease and how to treat it, and do so far more sensitively than any male physician. In 'Sex in Mind and Education: A Reply', Garrett Anderson's authority rests on this blend of medical training and female intuition.

Citing Maudsley's warning about the need for women to be wary of their 'special physiological functions,' she argues that 'it is difficult to understand what is meant, considering that in adult life healthy women do as a rule disregard them almost completely' (Garrett Anderson 1874, p. 585). She exposes the classism of Maudsley's theories, noting that 'among poor women, where all available strength is spent upon manual labour, the daily work goes on without intermission, and, as a rule, without ill effects' (Garrett Anderson 1874, p. 585). Thousands of women did not have the luxury to be mindful of their delicate constitutions and were living proof that menstruation is a normal physiological process. Garrett Anderson remarks that 'experience justifies a confident opinion that the cases in which it seriously interferes with active work of mind or body are exceedingly rare' (Garrett Anderson 1874, p. 586). In 'women of good health, the natural recurrence of this function is not recognised as causing anything more than very temporary *malaise*, and frequently not even that' (Garrett Anderson 1874, p. 586). As an educated woman whose living required her to do a great deal of intellectual and physical work, Garrett Anderson was uniquely qualified to write of this experience. Her own life, as both a mother and practicing physician, was more than reasonable proof that Maudsley's theories were unfounded. Such experience taught that menstruation must not be pathological, but Garrett Anderson also posits a medical explanation for why this may be so.

She suggests that if 'the demand made upon the nutritive processes' of the nerves is 'less in women than in men,' then 'nutrition is thus continually a little in excess of what is wanted by the individual, and there is a margin ready for the demand made in childbearing' (Garrett Anderson 1874, p. 585). Menstruation is therefore the female body ridding itself of the 'surplus nutritive material' and consequently causes 'no loss of vigour to the woman' (Garrett Anderson 1874, p. 586). Like Maudsley, Garrett Anderson draws on theories of energy conservation, but her experiential evidence leads her to an opposing conclusion. 'Sex in Mind and Education: A Reply' thus shakes the certainty of Maudsley's reasoning. For Garrett Anderson, there was no automatic connection between co-education and female mental illness, as there was no evidence, either experiential or clinical, that healthy women suffered from intellectual work.

Despite Maudsley's best efforts, change was already well underway in the higher education sector at this time. In mid-May, barely a month after his original article appeared and a week after Garrett Anderson's response was published, the University of London passed a vote in favour of allowing women entry to degree examinations. This was a major success in the campaign for female higher education and it only added fuel to the fire in the debate over 'Sex in Mind and in Education.' The *Examiner* now entered into the fray again with 'University Degrees for Women,' an article published in its 'Politics and Social Comments' section on 16th

May 1874. The article was written by Eliza Orme, who would go on to become the first woman to earn a law degree in Britain and who was one of the first nine women to earn the University of London's Certificate of Proficiency in 1869. As political commentary, the short-form piece is very different in tone to the correspondence offered in earlier numbers of the periodical and it demonstrates how Maudsley's theories had become entangled in current affairs. As a professional woman herself, Orme was resolutely pro-reform and the article begins by celebrating 'the vote in favour' of widening female access to higher education (Orme 1874, p. 508). Orme then lists the arguments commonly heard against 'change in the position of women' (Orme 1874, p. 508). Dismissing the majority, she argues that 'the statement which really deserves attention is the alleged incapacity of women for hard study,' the 'physiological aspect' of which Maudsley had recently discussed in the *Fortnightly Review* (Orme 1874, p. 508). She rejects his claims as 'utterly inconclusive' and irrelevant, particularly as the changes proposed by the University of London included none of the 'vexed questions of mixed classes' he raised about co-education (Orme 1874, p. 508). Orme does not cover the medical details of the case, but she takes a practical view of the subject: 'many women must work,' and if anything, being 'already handicapped in the race,' a degree will only assist them in the work they are 'obliged to do' (Orme 1874, p. 508). She therefore joined her fellow women respondents in refusing to engage with the panic Maudsley was attempting to stir, speaking as she could with assurance of her own capability for intellectual work.

The rapid and varied female response to Maudsley's article is striking. That so many female writers replied to the *Fortnightly* essay, in advance of any male correspondents, illustrates how actively women were involved in thinking about these issues. The debate is representative of the disputes over women's mental, emotional, and physical capacities that were happening across multiple discourses in the mid-nineteenth century. The women's movement was in full swing at this time and Garrett Anderson and Jex-Blake are its representatives here, both famously involved in campaigning for women's entry into medicine. Yet there were also women like Orme, quietly supportive of change and leading a life which reflected these views, and H.T., who resisted the interference of an overbearing and patriarchal medical profession. However, the discussion is unusual in its focus on the physiology of women's bodies and minds. The barriers to female participation in professional literature at this time meant that such dialogue had been, for the most part, invisible (both to contemporary readers and us as historians). With a wider audience and greater variety of literary forms, the non-specialist press gave women a voice and acted as a platform from which they could publicly contest male medical authority. This increased access to debate and expanded the parameters of medical discussion to include and validate women's own experiences of their mental and physical health.

It is significant, however, that none of these women challenged the centrality of reproduction to the female body or female identity. By the 1870s, psychiatry had firmly established that women's reproductive systems were in intimate sympathy with their minds. It is possible that the scientific authority of these theories, as well as the weight of centuries of ideology which supported them, made any alternative concept of female nature inconceivable. Although Garrett Anderson, Jex-Blake, H.T., and Orme challenged Maudsley's views in part, they were really arguing about the degree of impact. Whether refuting the belief that pathological change could happen in otherwise healthy women, or assuring the reader that women were capable of being in charge of their own menstrual health, these writers simply suggested that their sex could succeed *despite* the handicap of their physiology. Whichever shape the argument took, female reproductive capacity remained essential to the concept of womanhood and any discussion about women's abilities. To be a woman was to be a potential mother, with all that role entailed.

The Conservative Backlash

Despite the relative caution of these female contributors, Garrett Anderson's reply to Maudsley provoked some indignant criticism in the conservative press and the debate gathered fresh wind as a result. Garrett Anderson was a high-profile woman who had constructed an organised and compelling argument in support of female education, and it was perhaps because of this that two sceptical writers now felt obliged to voice their disapproval. These new contributors were male voices, writing from a conservative, non-medical position. Their orthodox values were threatened by Garrett Anderson's article, which represented a source of progressive, female expertise that unsettled the status quo.

The first article to deal with the *Fortnightly* controversy was one entitled 'Sex in Education', published in the *Saturday Review* on May 9th, the number following the publication of Garrett Anderson's essay (Sex in

Education 1874). The *Saturday* was a weekly periodical that positioned itself between the classic quarterlies and monthly magazines, addressing critical issues and providing debate on the business of the day at a faster pace than these slower news cycles. Priced at six pence a number, it targeted an educated, upper-middle-class readership and was notorious for its reactionary attitude (Bevington 1941; Fraser et al. 2003; Tilley 2009). In contrast to the *Fortnightly*, the *Saturday* had a policy of anonymous contribution that allowed it to cultivate a unified editorial voice of lofty respectability. The article in question was no exception to this rule. Like all other contributions to the periodical, 'Sex in Education' is unsigned. Nonetheless, the author's use of exclusionary pronouns and tendency to separate the narrative voice from female concerns gives the text a masculine tone. In any case, the writer readily adopts the *Saturday*'s condescending style to argue against co-education.

This tone is unsurprising as, unlike the *Examiner* and *Fortnightly*, the *Saturday Review* adhered to a socially conservative set of values. It strongly opposed the women's movement and, in the preceding years, had famously published Eliza Lynn Linton's essays lampooning emancipated women, including the controversial 'Girl of the Period' (Linton 1868). 'Sex in Education' opens by dismissing the need for debate on the matter at all. The writer laments that 'there seems to be much less difference between the disputants than might at first sight be supposed; and therefore very little reason, except the irritating nature of all disputes about women's rights, for the importation of any hostile spirit into the matter' (Sex in Education 1874, p. 585). Seemingly without any awareness of the irony of the situation, the writer then launches into what is quintessentially an opinion piece. Unlike the extended compositions of the more traditional reviews, the quicker publication schedule of the *Saturday* meant that it tended to offer short-form articles. The topical nature of the periodical, with its focus on up to the minute news and views, discouraged longer contributions and reasoned think-pieces in favour of snappy reporting. 'Sex in Education' therefore avoids debating the theoretical or physiological details of the issue and is almost entirely polemic. This style is suggestive of a lay author and the article gives some indication of how Maudsley's ideas were received by the general public.

Although agreeing that the current educational system is 'superficial and often most foolish,' and that 'women ought to learn more,' the author argues that this does not mean that they should 'go through the same course of study independently of any consideration of their different physical constitutions' (Sex in Education 1874, p. 585). The author's assumptions about these physical differences demonstrate the pervasiveness of gendered beliefs about the female body and mind at this time, even outside of the medical profession. Conceding that only time will tell if women will suffer from co-education, the writer insists that 'the presumption appears to us to be the other way,' though it is the 'tendency of feminine reformers' in general to 'overlook this obvious and very important fact' (Sex in Education 1874, p. 585). What exactly these facts and presumptions are, the author does not detail, but we can infer from the context of the article that he means women's reproductive capacities and their impact upon the female mind. Gendered theories about the female brain had already become common knowledge to the extent that, without explicitly discussing physiology, the author can assume that the reader is well versed in the biological handicaps of women. 'Sex in Education' thus demonstrates how the lay public could already claim authority over psychiatric knowledge at this time. This author, who was most likely not medically trained, could speak with the self-assurance of an expert and expect other members of the public to listen. Significantly, the author's misogynistic rhetoric reveals how gendered ideologies supported the mind doctor's views and may have promoted their acceptance. The ready adoption of such theories of female madness was no doubt due in large measure to the fact that they reinforced existing ideologies about women's place in society. As the author remarks, educating women in the same way as men simply does not make sense, given that they are the 'more docile and less vigorous sex' (Sex in Education 1874, p. 586).

The next contribution to the debate, 'Sex in Mind and Education: A Commentary', appeared in the June number of *Blackwood's Edinburgh Magazine*, and relied heavily on these gendered assumptions to denounce co-education (Cowell 1874). *Blackwood's* was a monthly miscellany known for its literary content. Costing two shillings and sixpence, it targeted readers of the same social class as the *Fortnightly*, though of a much more conservative ilk. Its topical articles focused on contemporary political issues, and the controversy between Maudsley and Garrett Anderson was just the sort of news it was likely to report on (Finkelstein 2002, 2009; Coyer 2017). Like the *Saturday* article, the authorial voice of 'A Commentary' is male. Although the article was published anonymously (as was the periodical's custom), the Wellesley Index identifies the author as Herbert Cowell, a barrister who wrote eighty-six articles for *Blackwood's* between 1873 and 1900. As a regular contributor to the magazine, he wrote mostly on politics or political-social issues. That someone of his profession would do so was not unusual. The writing no doubt supplemented his income from the law and his access to the courts made him a valuable source of information on these topics, not to mention the fact that his own personal values appear to have aligned with the publication's editorial stance. However, Cowell had rather surprising family connections, for he was married to Alice Garrett. Daughter of Newson Garrett, she was the sister of two very famous women: Elizabeth Garrett Anderson and Millicent Garrett Fawcett (Whittaker 1949). Cowell was therefore the brother-in-law of the very author he was disparaging. Given his connections, it is striking that his article took such a hard line on the women's rights movement and its campaigners. His commentary is a ferocious critique of his own sister-in-law's views; Cowell evidently had passionate opinions about female education, which he was willing to defend even above family loyalties.

Cowell mocks Garrett Anderson for ignoring what he calls 'the most elementary rules of physiological science,' it being an 'obvious truth' that women need to be cautious of their mental and reproductive health (Cowell 1874, p. 739). Female physiological inferiority is so taken for granted that even Maudsley is upbraided for failing to tell us 'something new as well as something true' (Cowell 1874, p. 743). After all, Maudsley was simply voicing 'what we all knew before [...] that women cannot have the same aims as men' (Cowell 1874, p. 744). Of all the articles discussed here, Cowell constructs the most explicit link between Victorian gendered social ideology and women's mental unfitness. He repeatedly refers to binary gender roles as a physiological fact. Linking co-education to the disruption of women's domestic duties and moral collapse, he argues that proposals for female higher education 'cannot be generally accepted without unsettling the relations between the sexes, and overturning the foundations of domestic morality' (Cowell 1874, p. 739). Cowell also uses religiously loaded language to describe the harm caused by women who disobey the laws of nature and the punishment that will befall them for disregarding their sex. Since the 'time of Eve,' he asserts, differences of sex have determined the mental qualities of men and women, and these are 'manifestly intended by nature to fit a woman for maternal duties' (Cowell 1874, pp. 744–745). Cowell therefore believes that education should develop the 'real capacities' of 'true womanhood,' or, in other words, the 'civilising' and 'elevating influences' which 'women hold in trust' for society (Cowell 1874, pp. 747–749). He thus supports Maudsley's view that co-education will have grave consequences for the human race and illustrates how existing social norms encouraged acceptance of psychiatric theories about gender.

As these responses demonstrate, Maudsley's theories about the female mind fitted seamlessly into a pre-existing worldview in which women were first and foremost reproductive beings. Reading and responding to Maudsley in the non-specialist press, lay people could utilise his clinical arguments to maintain the patriarchal status quo. These articles make it clear that there were many individuals who were not happy with women's changing place in society. Aside from the personal views of these authors, *Blackwood's* and the *Saturday* catered to a readership supportive of articles of this nature. By opening clinical concepts to general discussion and debate, Maudsley merely gave these writers the tools to think about the inferiority of the female mind from a medical perspective. Through publishing in the non-specialist press and applying these concepts to a social problem, he made psychiatry vulnerable (like other forms of science during this period) to popularisation in service against women's emancipation. Maudsley's article and the above responses thus expose how reciprocal action between medicine and ideology reinforced entrenched concepts of femininity.

Conclusion

The debate came to an end when the *Westminster Review* revived the topic for the last time in October 1874, offering a final challenge to Maudsley's way of thinking. The periodical's lead article, 'American Women: Their Health and Education' (1874), covered the debate around Edward Clarke's text, which had prompted Maudsley's essay. In line with the *Westminster*'s progressive intellectualism, the article wholeheartedly supported both co-education and female physicians in a decidedly forward-thinking fashion. Yet the writer had very little to say about Maudsley, only remarking that he 'repeats and re-enforces with but little variation' Clarke's words and that their shared ideas are 'believed to be groundless by other medical authorities' who have a 'special knowledge of the subject in question'—namely, women doctors (American Women 1874, p. 461). This is significant, for in championing female medical expertise above that of Maudsley and other male mind doctors, the writer demonstrates that women's claim to knowledge of and authority over their own bodies and minds was beginning to be taken seriously, at least by those outside of the profession.

Ironically, it was Maudsley's article and the ensuing debate that gave women the opportunity to respond to medical ideas about their minds and to define for themselves what their abilities were, both mental and physical. As Trevor Turner has shown, Maudsley's strategy of publishing 'Sex in Mind and in Education' in the non-specialist *Fortnightly Review* was successful in regard to his personal ambitions. The private practice he built proved 'extraordinarily lucrative,' enabling him to leave a sizable bequest on his death for the building of a mental hospital in his name (Turner 1988, p. 175). However, Maudsley also inadvertently created a space for others to challenge and critique his views. His essay gave the public a medical language and framework for thinking about women's role in society, but contrary to his intentions, writers used it to both prove and disprove the need to preserve gender norms. The general periodical press facilitated a wide response to his article, demonstrating how genre and market audience fundamentally affected how psychiatric theories on the female mind were defined and utilised. The non-specialist press treated women's mental health very differently to the clinical textbooks of Maudsley's colleagues.

References

Unpublished Sources

Elston, Mary Ann C. 1986. Women Doctors in the British Health Services: A Sociological Study of their Careers and Opportunities. PhD thesis: University of Leeds. https://etheses.whiterose.ac.uk/247/. Accessed 31 December 2024.

Thomson, Elaine. 1998. Women in Medicine in Late Nineteenth and Early Twentieth-Century Edinburgh: A Case Study. PhD thesis: University of Edinburgh, 1998. http://hdl.handle.net/1842/6903. Accessed 31 December 2024.

Published Sources

Bersohn, Leora. 2009. Examiner (1808–1881). In *Dictionary of Nineteenth-Century Journalism in Great Britain and Ireland*, ed. Laurel Brake and Marysa Demoor, 211–212. Ghent: Academia Press.

Bevington, Merle M. 1941. *The Saturday Review, 1855–1868: Representative Educated Opinion in Victorian England.* New York: Columbia University Press.

Brake, Laurel. 2000. The *Westminster* and Gender at Mid-Century. *Victorian Periodicals Review.* 33: 247–272.

Bright, Benjamin. Women and the Scottish Universities. *Examiner.* 3457: 451–452.

Brock, Claire. 2008. Elizabeth Garrett Anderson and the Professionalism of Medical Publicity. *International Journal of Culture Studies* 11: 321–342. https://doi.org/10.1177/1367877908092588.

Brown, Michael. 2011. *Performing Medicine: Medical Culture and Identity in Provincial England, c.1760–1850.* Manchester: Manchester University Press.

Burstyn, Joan N. 1980. *Victorian Education and the Ideal of Womanhood.* London: Croom Helm.

Cantor, Geoffrey, and Sally Shuttleworth, eds. 2004. *Science Serialised: Representations of the Sciences in Nineteenth-Century Periodicals.* Cambridge: MIT Press.

Clarke, Edward. 1873. *Sex in Education; or, a Fair Chance for the Girls.* Boston: J. Osgood & Company.

Cooter, Roger, and Stephen Pumphrey. 1994. Separate Spheres and Public Places: Reflections on the History of Science Popularisation and Science in Popular Culture. *History of Science* 32: 237–267. https://doi.org/10.1177/007327539403200301.

Cowell, Herbert. 1874. Sex in Mind and Education: A Commentary. *Blackwood's Edinburgh Magazine.* 115: 736–749.

Coyer, Meghan. 2017. *Literature and Medicine in the Nineteenth-Century Periodical Press: Blackwood's Edinburgh Magazine, 1817–1858.* Edinburgh: Edinburgh University Press.

Crowther, M. Anne., and Marguerite Dupree. 2007. *Medical Lives in the Age of Surgical Revolution.* Cambridge: Cambridge University Press.

Csiszar, Alex. 2018. *Authorship and the Politics of Knowledge in the Nineteenth Century.* Chicago: Chicago University Press.

Davis, I. P. 1883. Hygiene for Girls. *Golden Hours: A Monthly Magazine for Family and General Reading.* 177: 593–597.

Dawson, Gowan, Richard Noakes, and Jonathan R. Topham. 2004. Introduction. In *Science in the Nineteenth-Century Periodical: Reading the Magazine of Nature*, ed. Geoffrey Cantor, et al., 1–36. Cambridge: Cambridge University Press.

Dawson, Gowan, Bernard Lightman, Sally Shuttleworth, and Jonathan R. Topham, eds. 2020. *Science Periodicals in Nineteenth-Century Britain: Constructing Scientific Communities.* Chicago: Chicago University Press.

Easley, Alexis, Clare Gill, and Beth Rodgers, eds. 2019. *Women, Periodicals and Print Culture in Britain, 1830s–1900s*. Edinburgh: Edinburgh University Press.

Elston, Mary Ann C. 2017. Elizabeth Garrett Anderson (1836–1917). In *Oxford Dictionary of National Biography*. https://doi-org.liverpool.idm.oclc.org/ https://doi.org/10.1093/ref:odnb/30406. Accessed 31 December 2024.

Fielding Blandford, George. 1865. Acquitted on the Grounds of Insanity. *Cornhill Magazine*. 12: 426-440.

Finkelstein, David. 2002. *The House of Blackwood: Author-Publisher Relations in the Victorian Era*. University Park: Pennsylvania State University Press.

Finkelstein, David. 2009. *Blackwood's Edinburgh Magazine* (1817–1980). In *Dictionary of Nineteenth-Century Journalism in Great Britain and Ireland*, ed. by Laurel Brake and Marysa Demoor, 60. Ghent: Academia Press.

Fraser, Hilary, Stephanie Green, and Judith Johnston, eds. 2003. *Gender and the Victorian Periodical*. Cambridge: Cambridge University Press.

Garrett Anderson, Elizabeth. Sex in Mind and Education: A Reply. *Fortnightly Review*. 15: 582–594.

Hack Tuke, Daniel. 1877. Modern Life and Insanity. *Macmillan's Magazine*. 37: 130-140.

Hack Tuke, Daniel. 1878. Broadmoor, and our Criminal Lunatics. *Macmillan's Magazine*. 38: 137-142.

H.T. 1874. Sex in Education. *Examiner*. 3455: 399-400.

Jex-Blake, Sophia. 1874. Sex in Education. *Examiner*. 3457: 457.

Lightman, Bernard. 2016. Popularizers, Participation and the Transformations of Nineteenth-Century Publishing: From the 1860s to 1880s. *Notes and Records*. 70: 343–359. https://doi.org/10.1098/rsnr.2016.0029.

Linton, Eliza Lynn. 1868. Girl of the Period. *Saturday Review*. 25: 339–340.

Macintyre, Iain, and A. Munro. 2015. The Monro Dynasty and their Treatment of Madness in London. *Neurosciences and History* 3: 116–124.

McIntyre, Neil. 2014. *How British Women Became Doctors: The Story of the Royal Free Hospital and Its Medical School*. Croydon: Wenrowave Press.

Maudsley, Henry. 1867a. *The Physiology and Pathology of the Mind*. London: Macmillan & Co.

Maudsley, Henry. 1867b. On Some of the Causes of Insanity. *Journal of Mental Science*. 12: 488–502.

Maudsley, Henry. 1871a. Insanity and its Treatment. *Journal of Mental Science*. 17: 311–334.

Maudsley, Henry. 1871b. *Body and Mind: An Inquiry into their Connection and Mutual Influence, Specifically in Reference to Mental Disorders, Being the Gulstonian Lectures for 1870, Delivered before the Royal College of Physicians*. London: Macmillan.

Maudsley, Henry. 1874. Sex in Mind and in Education. *Fortnightly Review.* 15: 466–483.

Moulds, Alison. 2021. *Medical Identities and Print Culture, 1830s–1910s.* Cham: Palgrave Macmillan.

Nash, Sarah. 2010. What's in a Name?: Signature, Criticism, and Authority in the *Fortnightly Review. Victorian Periodicals Review* 43: 57–82. https://doi.org/10.1353/vpr.0.0108.

On Some Affections Incidental to Women- Hysteria. 1855. Reynold's Miscellany of Romance. *General Literature, Science, and Art.* 15: 324.

Orme, Eliza. 1874. University Degrees for Women. *Examiner* 3459: 508.

Peterson, Jeanne M. 1994. Medicine. In Victorian Periodicals and Victorian Society, ed. by J. Don Vann and Rosemary T. Van Arsdel. 22–44. Aldershot: Scholar Press.

Rowold, Katharina. 1996. *Gender and Science: Late Nineteenth-Century Debates on the Female Mind and Body.* Bristol: Thoemmes Press.

Rowold, Katharina. 2011. *The Educated Woman: Minds, Bodies, and Women's Higher Education in Britain, Germany, and Spain, 1865–1914.* New York: Routledge.

Rylance, Rick. 2004. 'The Disturbing Anarchy of Investigation': Psychological Debate and the Victorian Periodical. In *Culture and Science in the Nineteenth-Century Media*, ed. Louise Henson, et al., 239–250. Aldershot: Ashgate.

Savage, George Henry. 1918. Henry Maudsley. *Journal of Mental Science.* 64: 117–123.

Schofield, Alfred T. 1888a. Inside a Brain. *Leisure Hour.* 1: 263-270.

Schofield, Alfred T. 1888b. A Bad Headache. *Leisure Hour* 1: 831-834.

Schofield, Alfred T. 1889. Nervousness and Hysteria. *Leisure Hour* 1: 412-415.

Schofield, Alfred T. 1899. *The Unconscious Mind.* London: Hodder & Stoughton.

Schofield, Alfred T. 1904. *Unconscious Therapeutics, or, the Personality of the Physician.* London: J & A Churchill.

Schofield, Alfred T. 1905. *The Management of a Nerve Patient.* London: J & A Churchill.

Scull, Andrew. 1979. *Museums of Madness: The Social Organisation of Insanity in Nineteenth-Century England.* London: Allen Lane.

Scull, Andrew. 1993. *The Most Solitary of Afflictions: Madness and Society in Britain, 1700–1900.* New Haven: Yale University Press.

Scull, Andrew, Charlotte MacKenzie, and Nicholas Hervey. 1996. *Masters of Bedlam: The Transformation of the Mad-Doctoring Trade.* Princeton: Princeton University Press.

Sex in Education. 1874. *Saturday Review* 37: 584–586.

Shail, Andrew. 2010. Neurology and the Invention of Menstruation. In *Neurology and Modernity: A Cultural History of Nervous Systems, 1800–1950*, ed. Laura Salisbury and Andrew Shail, 59–80. Basingstoke: Palgrave Macmillan.

Showalter, Elaine. 1987. *The Female Malady: Women, Madness, and English Culture, 1830–1980*. London: Virago.

Shuttleworth, Sally, and Berris Charnley. 2016. Science Periodicals in the Nineteenth and Twenty-First Centuries. *Notes and Records.* 70: 297–304. https://doi.org/10.1098/rsnr.2016.0026.

Small, Helen. 2003. Liberal Editing in the *Fortnightly Review* and the *Nineteenth Century. Publishing History.* 53: 75–96.

Tilley, Elizabeth. 2009. *Saturday Review* (1855–1938). In *Dictionary of Nineteenth-Century Journalism in Great Britain and Ireland*, ed. Laurel Brake and Marysa Demoor, 557–558. Ghent: Academia Press.

Turner, Mark W. 2000. *Trollope and the Magazines*. Basingstoke: Palgrave Macmillan.

Turner, Mark W. 2009. Fortnightly Review (1865–1954). In *Dictionary of Nineteenth-Century Journalism in Great Britain and Ireland*, ed. Laurel Brake and Marysa Demoor, 227–228. Ghent: Academia Press.

Turner, Trevor H. 1988. Henry Maudsley: Psychiatrist, Philosopher, and Entrepreneur. In *The Anatomy of Madness: Essays in the History of Psychiatry*, vol. III, ed. W. F. Bynum, et al., 151–190. London: Routledge.

Turner, Trevor H. 2010. Henry Maudsley (1835–1918). *Oxford Dictionary of National Biography* 2024. https://doi.org/10.1093/ref:odnb/37747.Accessed31December.

Whittaker, Edmund T. 1949. Philip Herbert Cowell, 1870–1949. *Obituary Notices of the Fellows of the Royal Society.* 6: 375–384.

Women, American. 1874. Their Health and Education. *Westminster Review.* 46: 456–499.

CHAPTER 4

Within the Asylum: Patient Perspectives and Gendered Experience in the Crichton Royal Institution

As the preceding chapters have shown, whilst psychiatric theories about the female mind were gendered, these beliefs could be contested. The psychiatric profession operated under a core belief system in which reproductive biology was understood to be important to the medical treatment of insane women. However, these ideas were by no means stable. Although psychiatric textbooks were the authoritative site of knowledge within the profession, the theories and treatments they espoused did not always hold firm under scrutiny from outside observers, nor under the professional realities of patient overcrowding and varying levels of staff expertise. Returning to the asylum, it is possible to understand gendered theories as one of a complex set of factors influencing clinical decisions. This chapter examines the experiences of female psychiatric patients during the second half of the nineteenth century. It will investigate the treatment of insane women, seeking to understand how far gendered theories were translated into practice, and will uncover the perspectives of patients themselves.

It is notoriously difficult to locate patient voices in nineteenth-century medical archives. Since Roy Porter's (1985) call for patient-focused histories, scholars have sought to widen historiographical perspectives. In the history of psychiatry, Jonathan Andrews' work on Gartnavel Asylum has

M. Chapman, *Writing Women's Madness, 1845–1914*, Palgrave Studies in Literature, Science and Medicine,
https://doi.org/10.1007/978-3-031-97092-4_4

unearthed the voices of patients in case notes, which, he argues, 'provide the surest basis we have for understanding the changing nature of the experience of the insane in asylums since 1800' (Andrews, 1998, p. 255). Likewise, Michael Barfoot and Allan Beveridge (1990, 1993) and Allan Beveridge (1998) have explored the letters of patients in the Royal Edinburgh Asylum. Nevertheless, the evidence of patients' own words is limited and necessarily curated; what remains in the archive are the phrases, writings, and memorabilia which physicians chose to record. More recently, Cristina Hanganu-Bresch and Carol Berkenkotter (2012) and Robert Ellis et al. (2021) have demonstrated the importance of examining a variety of sources in the search for an authentic patient voice. Hazel Morrison (2013, 2016) has gained deeper understanding of patient experiences by reading doctor-authored narratives against the grain, through diligent analysis of the 'array of power structures, narrative conventions and spatial parameters' shaping the dialogue 'between patient and practitioner' (Morrison 2013, p. 21). Scholars such as Sara Newman (2011) and Sarah Chaney (2016) have also shown that patients sometimes had a degree of agency over their experiences within the institution. These studies establish that careful attention to the range of sources available in the asylum archive (including casebooks, patient letters, and admissions registers), makes it feasible to include the patient in the history of mental health treatment.

Literary scholars have identified another key location where the patient voice can be found: the asylum periodical. Published by a significant minority of institutions, these periodicals were produced by and for asylum populations across nineteenth-century Britain. Patients were the editors, contributors, and printers of asylum periodicals. They are therefore one of the largest resources of patient writing which is available to scholars. Jill McMillan (2008), Jonathan Glenn Tinnin (2019), and Mila Daskalova (2022) have demonstrated how asylum periodicals reflect the complexity of institutional life through recording first-hand the experiences and interests of patients. As Daskalova argues, what emerges from such publications is a 'plurality of voices that at some times sound harmoniously, while at others they clash, contradict, or seek to subvert or outpower each other' (Daskalova 2022, p. 22). However, Emily Jessica Turner has warned that a cautious approach is necessary: 'how accurately does this journal represent the 'true' experience of this asylum?' (Turner

2019, p. 29). As with clinical records, the 'obfuscation of [the] relationship between asylum, journal and patient' must be unpacked (Turner 2019, p. 29).

Scholars have yet to make use of both sets of valuable sources in their analysis of nineteenth-century asylums. Combining the study of clinical records and asylum periodicals presents the opportunity to examine multiple expressions of the patient voice in the same institution. The tensions between doctor-authored and patient-authored writing demonstrate that asylum life was often multifaceted, with patients experiencing varying levels of wellbeing, agency, and personhood. These sources are evidence of the shifting clinical and institutional factors which affected patients. As this book demonstrates, texts shaped both theory and practice in nineteenth-century psychiatry. In the asylum, case notes directed treatment practices (such as decisions over forced feeding, restraint, and rehousing), often impacting patients' daily lives. They were also disease-focused: patients were diagnostic subjects and cases to be managed. In contrast, the writing and publication of periodicals offered patients an avenue for recreation and personal expression. In asylum periodicals patients were individuals.

This chapter will read asylum records alongside patients' periodical writing, making visible the constraints of the text on the patient voice and revealing the complexity of female patient experiences in the asylum. Taking as a case study the Crichton Royal Institution in Dumfries, Scotland, this chapter will examine the lives of female patients during the decade from 1875–1885. This period covers a share of the superintendency of the three physicians who had command of the asylum in the nineteenth century, following the departure of the institution's first (and foundational) physician superintendent Dr W.A.F Browne, in 1857: Dr James Gilchrist (1858–1879), Dr James Adam (1880–1883), and Dr James Rutherford (1883–1907). The period therefore provides insight into a broad spectrum of the institution's management, whilst offering a relatively narrow scope which allows for in-depth exploration of the asylum archive.

Crichton Royal was a chartered, charitable asylum, intended for paying male and female patients (with an attached institution for paupers). It also had, from Browne's superintendency, a strong focus on moral management techniques. The asylum thus offered patients many entertainments, including the institution's own magazine: *New Moon; or Crichton Royal Institution Literary Register* (1844–1937). This chapter will first examine the lived experience of women patients at the CRI, through the evidence of the institution's admissions registers and casebooks. These records demonstrate that, although the classification and treatment of female patients in the CRI partially reflects the gendered theories presented in nineteenth-century psychiatric textbooks, these beliefs were not the primary factor in decisions made about patient care. Treatments were based on the asylum's moral management methodology and were designed to encourage appropriate patient behaviour, with quietness and industry perceived as signs of a rational mind. Nevertheless, the case notes do reveal the influence of doctors' personal beliefs about women, and patients' mental health was often measured against whether their behaviour met gendered social expectations, as well as clinical standards of cure.

The chapter will then turn to the writing of female patients in Crichton Royal's the *New Moon*. The asylum periodical was intended as one of a roster of activities available to patients under the institution's moral management methodology. Nevertheless, the *New Moon* became a valued part of asylum life for many patients and was an important vehicle for intellectual and personal expression. Significantly, the periodical gave women a platform of remarkable equality, not only on a par with male patients but also wider society. Women writers in the *New Moon* engaged in journalistic and literary work; something many would have found difficult to achieve outside of the institution. In fact, the periodical often published women's writing which directly engaged with contemporary debates about female emancipation. This chapter will take a closer focus on two female patients: Helen S. Traill and Lydia Cairns. Both women were chronic patients at the CRI. Elderly spinsters, they are often treated with contempt in the case notes. However, the *New Moon* provided the women with social status and intellectual fulfilment, and the pages of the magazine are a space where their individual voices can be heard.

These texts demonstrate that the experiences of female patients at Crichton Royal were nuanced and must be understood within the specific context of the institution. Clinical records shaped women's progress through the asylum and are reflective of the institution's professional methodology. In contrast, the *New Moon* facilitated women's exercise of their individuality through its distinctly non-clinical character. Both were important aspects of life at Crichton Royal for patients and practitioners alike.

The Diagnosis and Treatment of Female Patients at the CRI

Crichton Royal Institution was the last of Scotland's charitable, chartered Royal Asylums, opening in 1839. The existence of these seven institutions, dotted across Scotland's cities and major towns, predated lunacy reform. This system contributed to the delay of state intervention in the care of the insane, and the Lunacy (Scotland) Act was only passed in 1857 (Smith Clouston 1893; Cromhall Easterbook 1937; Scull 2011; Philo and Andrews 2017). Francis J. Rice has argued that the 'creation of a national, rationalised structure for the organisation of insanity in Scotland came twelve years after a similar body was instituted in England and Wales,' in part because the country had 'a far better developed, public charitable subscription sector than that which existed south of the border' (Rice 1981, p. 224). In the early nineteenth century, the Royal Asylums were just one of several different types of institution which housed the insane and many patients were cared for in the community. Nevertheless, the Royals 'bore the brunt' of care and, unlike poorhouses or infirmaries, were spaces dedicated to the insane (Rice 1981, p. 278).

They accepted a mixed class of patients, caring for paupers whilst also catering for what Rice terms the 'more rewarding' end of the market. Most 'offered a dual, class-demarcated service' (Rice 1981, p. 247). At Crichton Royal, demand was such that a new institution was built in 1849 specifically for pauper patients: the Southern Counties Asylum. The asylum was then split into two houses which (despite sharing a physician superintendent) were largely separate (McMillan 2008). By mid-century, the Crichton Royal Institution was exclusively for paying patients, though this included quite a large spectrum of the population, from artisans to gentlewomen. Eventually, institutional overcrowding made the need for new provision clear, and the state intervened. Following the legislation of 1857, 'a national co-ordinating body was established, a network of district institutions set up and a general tightening up of the existing law took place' (Rice 1981, p. 293). Both the Royals and district institutions were subject to inspection by the new Lunacy Commission, and patients were required to be certified before admission (from 1862 the CRI also took a small number of voluntary admissions).

In line with English legislation, Scottish law required strict record-keeping, including admissions certificates and a Register of Lunatics, Register of Restraint and Seclusion, and Register of Discharges and

Removals. The development of medical treatment for insanity (and anatomical-clinical medicine more broadly) gave record keeping greater clinical importance during this period. However, under the new Lunacy (Scotland) Act, such records also served an administrative purpose within the asylum (Lazenby Craig 1989, 1991; Risse and Warner 1992). The Registers were a method of monitoring patient populations, evidencing staff decision-making, and providing assurance of appropriate treatment practices and good management. These records thus illuminate the institutional response to the patient as well as indicate the clinical methodologies employed and are a vital source for tracking patients' experiences within the asylum. Reflecting shifting clinical and administrative attitudes, they also reinforced these practices in the institution. In fact, patients' lives were shaped by the clinical record from the moment of their arrival.

Classifying Female Insanity

A new patient at the CRI would have their certification reviewed, their history taken, and their physical condition examined. This data was collected for the Register of Lunatics, which recorded admissions to the asylum and categorised patients for appropriate management within the institution. The Register was a dedicated record book which contained a prefilled table including columns for the form and cause of mental disorder (Table 4.1). 'Form' indicated the class of insanity from which the patient was suffering and 'cause' the origin of their disease. These classifications were used to appoint patients to a room suitable to their condition. From the outset, the complex experiences and individuality of each patient were reworked into a diagnostic classification which decided the physical environment in which they would be housed. This was necessary for the efficient management of the institution and the protection of inmates (violent patients needed more supervision, for example). The process nonetheless instigated practitioners' conceptualisation of the patient as a clinical case and is a useful indicator of the factors which the institution considered important in the categorisation of the insane. The Register of Lunatics therefore played an important role in the reception and organisation of women patients at Crichton Royal and provides valuable evidence of how female insanity was perceived at the asylum.

Nineteenth-century psychiatric textbooks show that reproductive biology was a significant factor in the diagnosis and treatment of insane women, resulting in gendered disease categories. Yet, Crichton Royal's

Table 4.1 Example entry from Crichton Royal Register of Lunatics, 1881

Date of last previous admission (if any)	
No. in order of admission	1724
Date of admission	15th November 1881
Christian name and surname at full length	Ann Drummond or Wallace
Sex and class	F, private
Age	28
Condition as to marriage Single/Married/Widowed	Married
Condition of life and previous occupation	Farmer's wife
Previous place of abode	Shebtow Pasture, Penrith
County or parish to which chargeable	
By whose authority sent	J.F. Anderson, F.S
Dates of medical certificates and by whom signed	Dr M Leoch; J Borland, M.D. 15th Nov '81
Bodily condition	Fair
Name of disorder (if any)	Oedema of feet
Form of mental disorder	Lactational insanity
Supposed cause of insanity	Over nursing
Epileptic	
Congenital idiocy	
Duration of existing attack	
No. of previous attacks	
Age on first attack	28
Date of discharge, removal, or death	
Discharged removed/relieved/not improved	
Died	

Register of Lunatics indicates that this was only a secondary consideration in the classification of female patients. Between 1875 and 1884, 507 certified patients were admitted to the CRI.[1] 182 of these patients were female. Of these women, only 15 were recorded as suffering from a gendered form or cause of disorder. 3 were classed as having a specifically feminine form of insanity: 2 instances of climacteric insanity and 1 of lactational insanity. 2 of these 3 women were also recorded as having a reproductive cause; the cause of the remaining patient's disease is simply listed as 'unknown.' A further 12 women are listed as having a reproductive cause, without a feminine classification (CRI Register of Lunatics

[1] Records are incomplete. Patients from the end of 1884 and 1885 are missing from the series.

1839–1878 and 1878–1884). This is a vanishingly small number, with only 8.24% of the total female asylum population receiving a gendered diagnosis of some kind (Table 4.2).

With only 3 women classed as having a feminine form of disorder, these entries are statistical anomalies. Although more patients were assigned reproductive causes for their insanity, this was infrequent and is not indicative of a consistent clinical approach. It appears that for women of childbearing age, reproductive biology was only considered relevant to diagnosis when there was a clearly defined event which triggered an attack; such as the patient whose alcoholism was apparently caused by 'childbirth at sea' (CRI Register of Lunatics 1839–1878). 7 of the 15 cases associated with reproductive signs were elderly patients suffering from 'climacteric insanity' or 'change of life' (the menopause), indicating that the diagnosis may have been a useful explanation for the onset of symptoms in later life in women (CRI Register of Lunatics 1839–1878 and 1878–1884). Nevertheless, these patients still represent a small percentage of the total number of females admitted during this period. This data suggests that whilst reproductive biology was recognised as occasionally relevant to the diagnosis of women patients, mind doctors at the CRI did not work with a coherent theory of female insanity. In

Table 4.2 Gendered diagnoses given to female patients admitted to the Crichton Royal Institution, 1875–1884

Date	*Form of disorder*	*Cause of disorder*
1876	Melancholia	Change of life
1877	Dipsomania [alcoholism]	Childbirth at sea
1877	Delusional mania	Childbirth
1879	Melancholia	Change of life
1879	Climacteric insanity	Unknown
1881	Lactational insanity	Over nursing
1882	Mania	Suppression of menses
1882	Dementia	Change of life
1882	Melancholia	Childbirth
1882	Mania	Change of life
1882	Acute mania	Change of life
1883	Climacteric insanity	Climacteric
1883	Melancholia	Pregnancy
1884	Melancholia	Pregnancy
1884	Melancholia	Change of life

fact, the Register of Lunatics reveals that most patients at the CRI were classed as having one of five major forms of insanity: mania, melancholia, delusional insanity, dementia, or imbecility. This was a nosology based on disease presentation, rather than origin; patients were categorised according to observable behaviours and external symptoms, visible to the physician.

Increasing emphasis on anatomical and pathological knowledge in psychiatry made this approach out of date by the 1870s, as classifications were developed which considered the causes of mental disease. For example, David Skae's (1863) classification, developed in 1863 and recommended for use in casebooks by the Medico-Psychological Association (Halliday 2003), included categories like amenorrheal and syphilitic mania. Similarly, in his 1884 textbook *Insanity and Allied Neuroses*, George Henry Savage listed an 'ideal classification' which grouped forms of insanity under human developmental stage (such as 'insanity of adolescence') and recognised specific causes and symptoms (such as 'mania with conceit') (Savage 1884, pp. 10–11). Savage presented this system alongside a classification used 'for convenience,' which listed 13 different forms of insanity including 'hysteria-mania' and 'states of mental weakness-chronic mania and melancholia' (Savage 1884, pp. 11–12). Although Savage noted that 'any classification of insanity must necessarily be provisional [...] till our knowledge of mind in health and disease is greatly extended,' both his suggested systems emphasised aetiologically specific mental diseases (Savage 1884, p. 12).

However, at Crichton Royal aetiology was rarely used to classify a patient. The causes given in the Register of Lunatics are numerous, often being drawn verbatim from the statements provided by the certifying physician or the patient's relatives. Both physical and emotional causes are listed, such as 'heredity' and 'disappointment.' However, the origin of many patients' insanity is 'unknown' (CRI Register of Lunatics 1878–1884). Significantly, there is no pattern linking cause to the form of patients' disorder and there are only a handful of entries where an aetiologically specific form (such as lactational insanity) is given. Although reproductive biology was considered an important cause of female insanity, it was not thought to determine disease presentation; both male and female patients could experience manic or melancholic symptoms. Gendered signs were therefore not a major factor in the classification of insane women at the CRI, which was primarily driven by patients' behavioural profiles.

Crichton Royal's classificatory system resulted from the continued dominance of moral management methodologies at the institution. During the late nineteenth century, many Scottish asylums underwent a process of hospitalisation whereby medical and general hospital features were introduced, including facilities for clinical research and trained nurses. Emma Halliday has shown how the impetus for hospitalisation 'arose from debate between individual doctors' with 'Thomas Clouston [...] acknowledged as the leader' of the movement (Halliday 2003, p. 90). Both Clouston at the Royal Edinburgh and David Yellowlees at Gartnavel Asylum stressed somatic causes for mental disease (Andrews 1997). However, Crichton Royal's first physician superintendent, W.A.F. Browne, was a pioneer of moral management techniques and this ethos was maintained even after Browne resigned. Moral treatment focused on behaviour management in patient care and resulted in a decreased emphasis on biological factors in mental disease, including reproductive symptoms (Skultans 1975; Digby 1985; Charland 2007, 2012). As Halliday describes, 'moral approaches adopted psychological methods and occupation in the attempt to regulate reason and restore sanity' (Halliday 2003, p. 96).

Under a moral management methodology, classification was a tool for the asylum to encourage correct patterns of behaviour by organising patients into appropriate groups. W.A.F. Browne believed that patients should first be segregated by rate, as 'the pauper could not appreciate, nor prize, nor derive benefit from the refinement and delicacies essential to the comfort, and instrumental to the recovery of the affluent'; second, by stage of disease, so that the chronic 'may not prove injurious to those who are still capable of being influenced by moral impressions'; and third, by the 'disposition of the individual,' so that patients may positively affect one another by their complementary habits (Browne 1837, pp. 199–200). Browne argued that categorising patients in this manner would promote cure and ensure a smoother running institution.

Crichton Royal was modelled on Browne's theories and patients were housed in wards which corresponded to their classification and social class. The 1857 Royal Commission Report describes the accommodation for '120 patients of all classes,' 'consisting of eleven galleries' (Scottish Lunacy Commission 1857, p. 45). Rates at the CRI ranged 'from £30 to £350' per annum and separate accommodation was provided for patients paying different fees (Scottish Lunacy Commission 1857, p. 46): 'suites of two rooms [...] allowed to patients of the upper classes; a bed-room and the use of two public rooms to patients of the middle class; and a common dormitory and public room to patients of the lowest class' (Scottish Lunacy Commission 1857, p. 45). Further to this arrangement, patients were separated based on how disruptive they were: 'so far as is practicable, the patients are classified according as their intellect, sentiments, or propensities are affected, or according to the degree of fatuity' (Scottish Lunacy Commission 1857, pp. 48–49). As in all nineteenth-century asylums, patients were automatically divided by sex.

The classifications used at the CRI were therefore tied to decisions about patient housing, which supported a clinical methodology in which gendered theories of madness were of limited consequence. The moral treatment ethos of the CRI, alongside the administrative needs of the institution as a private facility, began to shape female patients' experiences from their earliest days in the asylum, far more than their sex. The classification of patients in the Register of Lunatics was instrumental to this process, initiating the transformation of individuals into diagnostic subjects (for example, as a manic or melancholic), as well as materially impacting patients' daily lives through the recording of data which determined their living quarters. To understand how women's experiences developed as they received treatment for their diagnosis, it is necessary to turn to the CRI casebooks, which provide the clinical record for each patient resident at the asylum.

Treating Female Insanity

Although there was no legal requirement to keep case notes under the Lunacy (Scotland) Act of 1857 (Halliday 2003), the CRI had done so since its foundation in 1839. Similarly to the Register of Lunatics, the casebooks follow a prescribed format. Each case was preceded by notes taken from the patient's Sherrif's Warrant. Required by all certified admissions from 1858, the Sherrif's Warrant was a standardised form, produced by the General Board of Commissioners in Lunacy. It contained a list of 20 statements giving an overall picture of the patient's person, health, and disorder (CRI Sherrif's Warrants 1838–1936). Following the Sherrif's Warrant came a dated diary of patients' care whilst at the asylum. This included information about the progress of their disease, any treatments received, and outcomes of the case. The casebooks are therefore a record of the asylum's clinical approach, revealing what signs of insanity doctors thought it important to notice, as well as how they attempted to cure their patients. Written from the perspective of the physician, they show how staff at the asylum perceived female patients and their symptoms.

For some women at Crichton Royal, reproductive biology *was* considered of pivotal importance in the cause, and therefore the diagnosis of, their disorder. Ann Drummond Wallace, age 28, was admitted for lactational insanity in April 1881. Unusually, a full history of the case was provided by relatives at admission. This is given in Ann's notes. The author writes that 'two years ago last February the first symptoms of mental derangement were noticed when Mrs Wallace had a miscarriage' (CRI Case Book Vol. 15 1876–1881). Ann recovered from this episode and was well until the 'present attack commenced last February about 9 months after the birth of her last baby which is now 18 months old' (CRI Case Book Vol. 15 1876–1881). The author thus draws clear connections between reproductive events in Ann's life and her disorder. After these events, Ann suffered insomnia, being 'very restless at night [...] one night she did not go to bed at all' (CRI Case Book Vol. 15 1876–1881). She also became very distressed, 'intending to harm herself' and trying to 'put her feet in the fire' (CRI Case Book Vol. 15 1876–1881). This contrasted with her natural disposition, which is said to be 'sweet, shy, and reserved' (CRI Case Book Vol. 15 1876–1881). The case history thus emphasises that Ann's erratic behaviour is directly caused by the reproductive changes she undergoes. After residing in the asylum for 6 months, Ann's symptoms lessened in intensity. However, she became 'very idle' and 'sometimes remains in bed' (CRI Case Book Vol. 16 1881–1885). The author records 'these symptoms appearing at the menstrual period,' which later ceased altogether (CRI Case Book Vol. 16 1881–1885). The patient's 'secondary dementia' is therefore also linked to reproductive causes and Ann's case is clearly one which mind doctors considered to be specifically feminine in nature (CRI Case Book Vol. 16 1881–1885).

However, this was not the case with all, nor even many, female patients. Even those given a reproductive cause or form of disorder were not always treated in a gendered fashion. Milicent Agnes Smallpiece, admitted in 1882 for acute mania caused by suppression of menses, was 'much troubled by delusions' and 'behaves in the most violent manner' (CRI Case Book Vol. 16 1881–1885). No mention of her menstruation is made in the case notes and treatments are aimed at lessening her violent behaviour: 'has had paraldehyde nearly every night and has slept a few hours nightly but not soundly' (CRI Case Book Vol. 16 1881–1885). Female patients classified under broader categories of disease presentation are likewise treated without reference to gendered signs. Catherine Hewison, 27, was admitted in 1878 for mania caused by over brain work and neuralgia. No mention is made at any time of reproductive causes or symptoms, and the case notes focus on the content of her delusions which related to 'food and her relations' (CRI Case Book Vol. 15 1876–1881). Another young woman, Cecilia Mary Boyee, admitted in 1882 at age 23 for dementia caused by insomnia, is simply noted as being 'slightly excited with delusions' and very 'unhealthy looking' (CRI Case Book Vol. 16 1881–1885). Although both these women are of childbearing age, there is no record of their reproductive history.

In fact, physicians sometimes dismissed patients' own claims of reproductive disturbance. Agnes Bryce Affleck was admitted to the asylum in 1879 at age 54, suffering from climacteric insanity. Delusions were the principal feature of her mental disease, with the certifying doctor stating that she 'believes her friends are continually plotting against her' and that she is always 'running to neighbours for protection from fancied enemies' (CRI Case Book Vol. 15 1876–1881). When settled at Crichton Royal, Agnes began to complain of her health: 'she is further very decided in her statements that she is suffering from some uterine disease' (CRI Case Book Vol. 15 1876–1881). However, the physician places these claims within Agnes's disease profile, viewing them as another delusion which 'so far has not been corroborated by any evidence' (CRI Case Book Vol. 15 1876–1881). He draws this conclusion even though Agnes has a 'pale unhealthy appearance' and is one of the few patients classified under a reproductive form of insanity (CRI Case Book Vol. 15 1876–1881).

These findings broadly reflect the patterns of diagnosis evident in the Register of Lunatics. Although attention is paid to reproductive symptoms in the notes of some women patients, this is not uniform across the female population. These cases, like that of Alice Bennett who 'has been insane since the birth of her child a fortnight ago,' can be linked to specific reproductive events: usually, childbirth, or the 'puerperal state' (CRI Case Book Vol. 15 1876–1881). Morag Allen Campbell has demonstrated that puerperal insanity was a diagnosis regularly used in Scottish asylums during the mid nineteenth century, accounting for 'approximately 7% of female admissions over the period 1835–60' at Dundee Asylum, and a similar percentage of 'female admissions to the Royal Edinburgh Asylum in 1846–64' (Allen Campbell 2016, p. 48). Although women at Crichton Royal are not often given this specific diagnosis there is marked attention to symptoms arising concurrently with, or directly after, the puerperal period. Hilary Marland has shown how puerperal insanity was a prominent diagnosis throughout the Victorian period, as the 'massive contravention of social norms [...] demonstrated by women suffering from puerperal mania was particularly shocking' (Marland 2004, p. 4). Studied by other medical disciplines such as neurology and obstetrics, the condition was thought to arise from the physical as well as mental trauma of birth. The social significance of the disease and its recognition within the wider medical community goes some way to explain the attention given to childbirth in patients' reproductive history, even though theories of female insanity were not widely applied at Crichton Royal.

Even female patients who experienced reproductive symptoms were not treated for them. Rather than addressing the physical or psychological consequences of patients' reproductive histories, the primary focus of the case notes is women's behaviour whilst at the asylum. Treatments aimed to improve unwanted or disruptive habits. Patients who refused to eat frequently met with the threat or actual use of the stomach pump (forced feeding), such as in the case of Agnes Affleck who 'refused food but when the stomach pump was given as an option to her eating her dinner she preferred the latter' (CRI Case Book Vol. 15 1876–1881). Those who were destructive in their habits were 'corrected' with punishments which induced behaviour modifications. Agnes, for example, became 'addicted to tearing her dress' and a 'strong canvas dress was put on for some days' to prevent this (CRI Case Book Vol. 15 1876–1881). Troublesome patients were also sometimes removed to other parts of the asylum, to ensure that they did not disturb other residents. Ann Drummond Wallace was housed in the infirmary following an attack of typhoid fever but became 'violent' and 'when her bowel moved she behaved most disturbingly, smearing herself and smearing everything around her' (CRI Case Book Vol. 16 1881–1885). Consequently, 'she was moved from this infirmary to the Low East and an official attendant put to watch her' (CRI Case Book Vol. 16 1881–1885). These transfers also served as a punishment for undesirable behaviour, relocating paying patients to less comfortable surroundings.

Reformed behaviour was a sign of patients' clinical progress. Quietness and industry were particularly encouraged, being considered a marker of mental health. After her time in the Low East, Ann improved and was able to return to her regular room. The case notes state that she 'has been in fair mental health, quiet and very industrious, a great help to the attendant in whose gallery she is' (CRI Case Book Vol. 16 1881–1885). The author also writes approvingly that Ann 'attends the amusements' provided by the asylum (CRI Case Book Vol. 16 1881–1885). Likewise, Milicent Smallpiece's condition is assessed on her ability to take part in the employments encouraged at Crichton Royal. In January 1884, the case notes record her sad propensity to sit 'all day tucked on a chair scarcely speaking and never working' (CRI Case Book Vol. 16 1881–1885). One year later she is somewhat improved, sometimes 'working and writing letters' (CRI Case Book Vol. 16 1881–1885). The degree to which the women engaged with the moral treatments offered at the asylum therefore signified their recovery or relapse. A cured patient was one who could follow the rules of the institution, undertake employment suitable to their social station and sex, and converse reasonably with their peers. These were key tenets of moral management methodology.

Scholars such as Vieda Skultans (1975), Emma Halliday (2003), and Sarah Chaney (2016) have emphasised the shunning of idleness in nineteenth-century moral treatment practices. Halliday has described how the 'engagement of patients in work was linked to the individual's recovery and discharge' (Halliday 2003, p. 108). Work was 'regarded to be both a therapeutic agent and a sign of recovery,' helping patients to get well and serving as a measure of their sanity (Halliday 2003, p. 108). Lorraine Walsh (2004), in her study of Dundee Royal Asylum, has demonstrated that these treatment practices were applied for private patients, as well as paupers. Walsh argues that the 'wholesale incorporation of the Protestant work ethic' into moral management methodologies connected respectability with activity, thus ensuring that even paying patients were encouraged to occupy themselves whilst at the asylum (Walsh 2004, p. 257). The 'increasing number of middle-class individuals who were entering the asylum as private patients on the lower and often subsidised rates of board' also limited the ideological discord between therapeutic occupation and patients' normal lives, as most would have been employed in some capacity outside of the institution (Walsh 2004, p. 258).

The epistemological emphasis on reproductive biology as a cause of female insanity was thus balanced by the specific clinical approach to the care of the insane, taken at Crichton Royal. Reading the case notes, it is evident that physicians at the CRI undertook the treatment of women patients on a behavioural basis, and did not perceive women's mental illness to be 'female insanity' in particular. This approach mirrored the classification of patients based on disease presentation and resulted from the moral management methodologies employed at the asylum. The importance of institutional factors in the treatment of insanity has been corroborated by research into patterns of diagnosis in other Victorian asylums. These studies indicate that there was significant variation in psychiatric practice during this period, with methodologies differing across institutions. Morag Allen Campbell's (2017) examination of puerperal insanity at Dundee Royal has presented evidence of the routine deployment of aetiologically specific, gendered diagnoses and treatments in subsections of the female asylum population, whereas Simon A. Hill and Richard Laugharne (2003) have demonstrated that from 1870–75 the broader categories of mania, dementia, and melancholia were employed almost exclusively at St Lawrence's asylum in Bodmin, Cornwall. The moral treatment practices of the CRI are further evidence of this differentiation and demonstrate that the treatment of female asylum patients must be understood within the wider context of continuing professional development in psychiatry.

Despite this, there is evidence of practitioners' gendered attitudes to women patients within the CRI casebooks. Written from the physician's perspective, the case notes include the author's reaction to patients' symptoms. Physicians' reactions to their female patients are frequently personal and value laden, stemming from their social expectations of appropriate female conduct. Under a moral management ethos, in which approved behaviour signified recovery, these beliefs shaped clinical perceptions of health and disease in women patients.

Curing Unfeminine Behaviour

As at other asylums in Britain during the nineteenth century, the CRI was administered via a hierarchy of staff, from the physician superintendent down to the servants. Although the superintendent directed the methodology of the asylum and was responsible 'generally for the care and treatment of the patients,' it was the more junior medical assistants who managed the day-to-day clinical practice (Jardine 1880). The medical assistants were (male) doctors, qualified under the 'terms of the Medical Act' (Jardine 1880). Their responsibility included all psychiatric and medical treatment of patients (general care and nursing was the duty of the unqualified attendants). To this end, the medical assistants visited their patients 'every morning' and 'personally report[ed] their condition to the Medical Superintendent' (Jardine 1880). They were also required to 'make special visits to the sick, the refractory, the recently admitted, or others requiring more particular attention' (Jardine 1880). Having such close knowledge of patients, it was also their responsibility to 'keep in good order all legal Registers and Books, and such others as may be deemed necessary by the Board of Directors or Medical Superintendent' (Jardine 1880). This included the keeping of the casebooks.

The authors of the case notes were therefore those practitioners who had most intimate contact with the asylum's patients and the notes reflect a personal element to patient care. Significantly, the medical assistants frequently employed language suggestive of their emotional response to the patient. Emotive terms such as 'vile', 'peculiar', and 'outrageous' are used to describe patients' behaviours, introducing a moral register into the clinical domain (CRI Case Books Vol. 15 1876–1881 and Vol. 16 1881–1885). These personal judgements percolate through the clinical data of the reports, making it possible to identify where physician's preconceived beliefs informed their care. This is notably different to the published psychiatric case history, discussed in Chapter 2 of this book. The case histories in nineteenth-century psychiatric textbooks follow an ordered narrative, primarily make use of clinical language, and provide a coherent, representative example of disease type. Such published histories were an after-the-fact selection and reordering of notes made in situ, making sense of hundreds of pages of dense asylum casebooks. In contrast, the Crichton Royal case notes are raw data and perhaps better reflect the realities of institutional life, where familiarity and frustrations developed between patient and physician.

It is the discursive quality of the case notes which allows for the personal voice of the clinician to come to the fore, their unstructured, diary-like form providing space for the expression of opinion alongside the recording of clinical facts. Prior to 1885 and the introduction of printed forms for the Sherrif's Warrants, the casebooks were simply bound volumes of lined paper, offering medical assistants the freedom to comment on each case as they pleased. The information recorded in the case notes differs between patients and is seemingly dictated by the interest of individual medical assistants. Although entries are dated, they are often irregular, with gaps of many months in the cases of long-term patients. The notes are written in lengthy prose, usually in the present perfect or present perfect continuous. They thus employ a reflective tone, as if the author's thoughts are occurring to him during conversation with a colleague. This was a form which evidently encouraged the author to record his personal feelings on the case, and many include the clinician's undisguised reaction to his patients' symptoms. Significantly, the male medical assistants at Crichton Royal expressed distaste with unfeminine and unladylike behaviour from their female patients, often reproving those whose behaviour failed to meet standards of propriety.

Bad language was particularly frowned upon and physicians responded to this behaviour with disgust. Milicent Agnes Smallpiece was a particularly intractable patient. 'Suffering from acute mania,' she was often violent and noisy (CRI Case Book Vol. 16 1881–1885). Milicent's case notes include regular entries describing her as 'chattering wildly and incoherently' and being 'exceedingly talkative' (CRI Case Book Vol. 16 1881–1885). This noisiness alone is clearly perceived as problematic, but the author also notes with disdain that 'her language is far from choice' (CRI Case Book Vol. 16 1881–1885). Milicent's volubility and rudeness is treated with drugs: 'she is having bromide of pot grd 15 [potassium, ground, 15 mg] three times a day and is now much quieter and more sensible' (CRI Case Book Vol. 16 1881–1885). Likewise, when Eliza Harvey was admitted in 1883 for delusional insanity following disappointment in marriage, she was upbraided for her use of 'shockingly bad language' (CRI Case Book Vol. 16 1881–1885). She became a chronic manic patient and remained resident at the asylum until 1917, continuing to use the 'vilest tongue' and 'most obscene language' (CRI Case Book Vol. 16 1881–1885). Mary Murray, admitted for recurrent mania, suffered from delusions. According to her medical assistant, these fancies were rendered 'still more ludicrous' by Mary's relating them 'in an uncouth patois' (CRI Case Book Vol. 15 1876–1881). Garrulity, loudness, monopolising conversation, and cursing were all considered undesirable in female patients and associated particularly with mania.

Obstinacy was also little tolerated and appears to have been profoundly irritating to medical staff. The case notes of Catherine Hewison reveal that, although 'very docile' when well, she began to show 'a considerable amount of obstinacy' from the onset of her illness (CRI Case Book Vol. 15 1876–1881). The author writes huffily that 'this young lady has been very capricious since admission' (CRI Case Book Vol. 15 1876–1881). Similarly, Margaret Hare, admitted in 1880 at 65, is described as 'very irritable' and a 'great nuisance' (CRI Case Book Vol. 15 1876–1881). Mary McVeigh, 50, was admitted in 1879 for mania but refused to engage with staff at all. The case notes record her 'childish obstinacy and whining objections to whatever is proposed for her benefit and comfort' (CRI Case Book Vol. 15 1876–1881). She 'continued to be obstinate' throughout her time at Crichton Royal, until she was 'discharged relieved'; though the author notes wryly that 'she is in much the same condition as when she came here' (CRI Case Book Vol. 15 1876–1881). For male medical practitioners, accustomed to a position of authority due to their class, sex and professional status, it must have been jarring to be rebuffed by female patients, many of whom would have been expected to submit to husbands and male relatives at home.

Indecent and erotic behaviour was also treated as a sign of insanity. Cecilia Mary Boyee's 'conversation is very unbecoming and quite unlike the usual,' particularly for a 23-year-old daughter of a reverend (CRI Case Book Vol. 16 1881–1885). Her behaviour is also described as 'outrageous,' a euphemism suggestive of a lack of sexual innocence perceived as uncouth in a young, single lady (CRI Case Book Vol. 16 1881–1885). Catherine Mary Butcher, age 35 at admission in 1877, suffered under delusions of a sexual nature, with a long standing 'tendency to obscenity' and recurring 'maniacal attacks characterised by eroticism' (CRI Case Book Vol. 15 1876–1881). During a previous stay in another asylum, she is said to have 'eloped with a groom' (CRI Case Book Vol. 15 1876–1881). Catherine's medical assistant describes with distaste how she frequently develops 'stories of an indelicate nature about those with whom she comes into contact' and imagines 'herself to be married to various persons and signing herself by their names' (CRI Case Book Vol. 15 1876–1881). The medical assistant notes that 'her conversation is very obscene at times' (CRI Case Book Vol. 15 1876–1881). In fact, this open sexuality is the primary feature of her disorder and Catherine exhibits few other symptoms of insanity. The explicit expression of sexual fantasy is such a severe contravention of social norms that it is indicative of a clinically significant loss of emotional control.

Although these behaviours are recorded in the case notes as markers of an unsound mind, the authors do not connect their remarks to specific psychiatric theories. There is no reference to the aetiology of such symptoms, or discussion of their pathology. Rather, these are behaviours which the medical assistants found personally offensive in female patients. Clair Scrine, in her study of nymphomania, describes how nineteenth-century diagnoses of the disorder 'lay with the sense in which the afflicted had acted 'indecently', or more accurately, in a manner contrary to 'middle class' sensibilities' (Scrine 2003, p. 110). Such 'class-specific expectations and beliefs about women's modesty and restraint' are at the heart of the medical assistants' disparaging comments which pepper the case notes (Scrine 2003, p. 110). Respectable middle-class women were passive, both sexually and in obeyance to the will of their male guardians (Vicinus 1972; Gorham 1982; Medus and Rendall 1989; Barret-Ducrocq 1991; Gleadle 2001). This was demonstrated through a quiet, meek demeanour directly at odds with the loud, reckless behaviour of CRI patients. Such behaviours excited scorn in the medical assistants because they contradicted ideologies of gender which emphasised women's modesty and innocence. Evidence that women *could* use bad language and act lewdly threatened the stability of these beliefs. This provoked a reaction in the assistants at the same time as those individuals attempted to explain the behaviours as evidence of mental imbalance. As Scrine notes, behaviours perceived as unhealthy were usually indicative of 'woman's loss of control' (Scrine 2003, p. 114).

Of course, the behaviours disliked by CRI medical staff were not only problematic because of the transgression of gender norms but were those most difficult to manage in an asylum setting. The loud, resistant, and obscene behaviours described above were disruptive to those around the patient, threatening the quiet order of the institution. Such behaviour contrasted with the decorum expected of patients under moral management. In female cases, a patient's ability to satisfy expectations clinically and socially (in line with doctors' gendered beliefs) was a measure of their sanity. Improvement is noted in Catherine Hewison's case, her physician writing that she 'is much more contented and less obstinate, she takes her food well—is industrious and promises well' (CRI Case Book Vol. 15 1876–1881). Although Margaret Hare is often violently emotional, the author notes approvingly that she is 'in general quite ladylike in her behaviours even when angry' (CRI Case Book Vol. 15 1876–1881). Similarly, Mary Murray is considered recovered as she is 'now very nice and agreeable' (CRI Case Book Vol. 15 1876–1881). Submission to professional (male) authority, willingness, and quietness are all positive attributes of both ideal womanhood and the recovering psychiatric patient.

The CRI casebooks reveal how women's lives at the asylum were shaped in part by the gendered beliefs of clinical practitioners but were nonetheless largely directed by the institution's moral management methodology. The asylum's clinical records, from the Register of Lunatics to patient case notes, were produced under this methodology, with the institution's administrative and clinical concerns in mind. In turn, they shaped physicians' medical practice and consequently the experiences of patients at the asylum. These records therefore provide useful insight into the CRI's clinical approach to female patients. However, women's stories are only told from the perspective of the institution and its staff. The Register of Lunatics erases all individuality in patients arriving at the asylum and the case notes tell little of women's experiences of mental illness from their own point of view. As in published case histories, the patient's voice rarely features in the case notes and any record of women's words is filtered by the medical assistant writing the entry. It is therefore important to turn to another record of asylum life at Crichton Royal: the institution's periodical.

Female Voices in the *New Moon*

A small but significant number of nineteenth-century British asylums produced their own periodicals, including the CRI. In fact, most asylum periodicals were published by institutions in Scotland, where both literacy rates and the percentage of the population engaged in publishing or related trades were high (Holligan 2024). Mila Daskalova's doctoral thesis, *Printing and Periodical Culture in the Nineteenth-Century Asylum* (2022), is currently the most comprehensive study of asylum periodicals available. Daskalova describes how the practice of creating and publishing these titles originated in the 1830s as a 'therapeutic instrument' (Daskalova 2022, p. 50). Usually 'written and edited at least partly by patients,' asylum periodicals were viewed by institutions as occupational therapy and were part of a wider moral management methodology (Daskalova 2022, p. 1).

This was certainly the case for Crichton Royal's periodical, which was founded by W. A. F. Browne in 1844 and intended as one of the therapeutic employments offered at the asylum (de Young 2015). Titled the *New Moon; or, Crichton Royal Institution Literary Register*, it ran until 1937 and was a regular feature of asylum life during the nineteenth century (McMillan 2008; Turner 2019). Browne planned for the *New Moon* to occupy patients' minds: the periodical was a '"mode of employing [...] dormant or valueless energies"' by redirecting them towards '"the amusement of the rest of the community."' (Glenn Tinnin 2019, pp. 121–122). Publishing and printing work may also have had direct relevance to patients at the CRI, who could conceivably have been employed in these local occupations prior to their stay at the asylum (Daskalova 2021). Similarly to the other opportunities for work and entertainment provided at Crichton Royal, the *New Moon* both gave patients practical skills and served a clinical purpose, promoting refinement of intellect and thus encouraging patients to develop the civilised thoughts and behaviours representative of mental health under the asylum's moral management ethos.

As Jill McMillan has noted, the periodical maintained a 'commitment to education and entertainment' through improving (though by no means light) content, suited to its therapeutic approach (McMillan 2008, p. 53). One of the earliest asylum periodicals, the *New Moon* helped to set the tone for the genre, which became a recognisable corner of the periodical market by mid-century. Described by Daskalova as 'miscellanies,' asylum periodicals shared a similar form and were usually of a literary and cultural character (Daskalova 2022, p. 1). They often featured 'humble poetry, discussions of current political and social topics, and essays on philosophical or scientific questions' (Daskalova 2022, p. 129). Through writing and reading of these subjects, patients could develop their capacity for reason and improve their mental health.

The *New Moon* was published in 4-page monthly numbers and was a miscellany with a literary leaning. It maintained a mix of poetry, fiction, drama, and topical articles, though its recurring features altered slightly to suit the changing fashions of the periodical market and tastes of its audience. Like other periodicals in the genre, it had a strong focus on the activities and writing of asylum residents. During the decade under consideration in this chapter, the *New Moon* primarily published original literary and journalistic work by CRI patients, who also printed the periodical on the Crichton Press. In addition, each number carried an editorial covering the asylum amusements from the preceding month, alongside a list of those planned for the coming weeks. From the 1880s onwards, puzzles and riddles were included, and reports of sports matches. These, too, were authored by patients.

The *New Moon* had numerous authors from within the patient population. In common with much of the nineteenth-century periodical market, most contributions to the *New Moon* were pseudonymous or anonymous. Nonetheless, it is possible to identify individual authors by their alias or initials. Between 1875 and 1885, there were 121 identifiable contributors to the periodical. This was approximately a quarter of patient admissions to the CRI during this period, which is a substantial portion of the asylum population, considering that there were many more contributors who remained anonymous. Not all patients would have been well enough to write for the periodical and it can therefore be assumed that many of those who were able to contribute did so. Many patients made multiple submissions to the *New Moon* during their time at the asylum, with three quarters of identifiable contributors publishing 3 or more times, and a core group of patients publishing on a regular basis with between 10 and 30 publications each over the 10-year period. Both male and female patients signed their contributions to the *New Moon* and at least 2 women are identifiable as part of the circle of regular contributors.

Crichton Royal's population thus enthusiastically participated in the magazine's production and the publication was an important part of patient life at the asylum. As Daskalova (2022) has shown, asylum periodicals often developed far beyond their therapeutic benefit. They were not only distributed amongst patients and staff, but sold 'outside their respective institutions, for profit,' the proceeds of which were intended to benefit the institution (Daskalova 2022, p. 2).[2] They were an important method of self-representation for asylum patients, both within the institution and to the outside world, and 'built and maintained communities both real and imagined' (Daskalova 2022, p. 3). In the *New Moon*, authors write proudly of their magazine and its readership. For example, in the January 1875 number, the editors 'beg to return our hearty thanks to our many friends, who have responded so liberally to our [Christmas] appeal' (Our Christmas Tree for 1874, 1875). There is also a sense of fraternity amongst the asylum population, for which the periodical is the collective voice. Important pieces of asylum news are regularly shared, including memorials for departed patients such as 'D.F.,' who had 'twenty years sojourn in our community' (In Memoriam D.F. 1875). Likewise, the monthly commentary on asylum amusements demonstrates fondness for certain patients, assumed to be recognisable to the reader. The December 1875 number reports on a party given by 'a lady resident, well known in our circle for her hospitality and the kind interest she displays

[2] Like other asylum periodicals during this period, the *New Moon* was intended for both an internal and external readership. Available on subscription, the periodical was priced in 1875 at 3d per number, or 3s for an annual subscription (3s 6d if subscribing by post). In February 1884 the price was lowered to 1d per number, or 1s annually (1s 6d by post).

in the happiness and welfare of all around her' (Amusements, &c, During the Past Month 1876).

However, although the *New Moon* was embraced by CRI residents as a valuable organ of their community, the therapeutic intentions of the institution necessarily meant that the periodical was a mediated space. As Emily Jessica Turner has argued, the *New Moon* was a product of 'collaboration, negotiation and exchange' between staff and patients (Turner 2019, p. 3), and is characterised by 'dialogue between the ideological impact of the asylum and an inmate-centric literary independence' (Turner 2019, p. 32). Such ideological tensions in the making of the periodical mean that a cautious approach must be taken in studying the publication as an authentic record of patients' unvarnished experiences. The *New Moon* was typically not an arena in which patients could express their psychopathology; symptoms of insanity would have been at odds with the therapeutic benefit expected from writing for the periodical.

Despite this, the moral management ideology which conflicted with the free expression of patients' unfiltered mental state also created a space where patients could regain their personhood. What Turner has described as 'the notion that "refinement" is equivalent to "wellbeing"' enabled patients to affirm their individuality through exercising their talents and expressing their interests (Turner 2019, p. 32). This philosophy encouraged patients to engage in diverse discussion and literary pursuits, so long as they were of a suitably intellectual and 'civilised' character. The content of the *New Moon* was broad in scope and patients expressed a range of views on a variety of topics. In 1876 alone, articles were published on art (F.M. 1876); psychology (On British Associationism 1876); travel (Erlana 1876); and current affairs (a satire imagining a matriarchal future with a disastrous government of women (A.C.M 1876)). The *New Moon's* literary and cultural focus, resulting from its moral management ethos, rendered its pages a distinctly non-clinical space, where patients transcended their status as mere cases in the asylum and became individuals with hobbies and political views.

In the *New Moon* women presented themselves as educated, informed, and capable. This was a part of asylum life where female patients could counter doctors' assumptions about both their mental health and their gender. In fact, the asylum periodical offered female patients a remarkable degree of agency. The periodical gave them a personal voice, a public face, and an intellectual platform, likely much wider than any available to them outside the asylum. The *New Moon* was a remarkably egalitarian occupation at the Crichton Royal, open to both sexes, and women were included in the civilising, intellectualising aims of the asylum's therapeutics. Female patients wrote on as varied topics as their male counterparts. Through the periodical, they were able to engage in journalistic and literary work, exercising poetic creativity and discussing not only institutional life but wider society. The *New Moon* thus allowed women to assert their personhood both as patients and as active and intelligent citizens.

This chapter will now discuss women's writing in the *New Moon*, taking as a case study female patients' discussion of women's emancipation during the 1870s, and focusing on the writing of two patients in particular: Lydia Cairns and Helen S. Traill. These cases show how the periodical enabled women to demonstrate an intellectually engaged social consciousness and, through this, to develop a voice entirely at odds with the disorder and disturbance presented in the CRI case notes.

Women Journalists, Women's Rights, and the Patient Voice

Female patients engaged in topical journalism on current affairs and from 1875–1880 content in the *New Moon* mirrored that seen in the wider periodical press, with a focus on the rights of women. Contemporaneous to the debate over Henry Maudsley's *Sex in Mind and in Education* (Chapter 3), female patients at Crichton Royal were participating in discussion about the role of women in society, women's education specifically, and the nature of femininity. 10 articles on these topics were published by women across 17 separate numbers of the periodical during this period.

It appears that the *New Moon's* editor did not censor patients' opinions on the topic. Crichton's female residents expressed a range of views in the periodical, demonstrating both conservative and progressive attitudes to women's rights. Some patients celebrated the new opportunities for women, such as the anonymous author who described her visit to the ladies' college in 'A Day at Girton', praising its laboratory 'full of scientific apparatus' and the 'spirit of genial hospitality' amongst its students (A Day at Girton 1880). In fact, one patient explicitly drew a connection between the success of the *New Moon* and its educated female contributors: 'A seeming custom 'tis to bow to the *New Moon*' but 'when, reflected, men see Girton there' (A Day at Girton 1880). The interesting and enlightened articles published by women in the periodical, enjoyed by all readers, would not be possible without the authors' increased access to education.

However, patients' contributions often revealed complex beliefs, as they struggled to reconcile entrenched ideologies with the shifting place of women in society. Hilda Evelyn Jane's lecture on 'Ladies, Would-Be's [sic], and Women,' published from May to September 1876, traced the fine distinctions in ladylike behaviour between different social classes and compared these to the true nature of woman as a '"help-meet for man"' (Jane 1876). Yet, the article ends with a rather tongue-in-cheek description of the ways in which women have 'atoned for the first great fault of the "mother of mankind"' (Jane 1876). They have:

> 'darned many pairs of man's stockings, put many a button on man's shirts, cooked him many a dinner, baked his bread, made his toast and tea, his porridge also; kept his house, cleaned it, washed his linens and woollens, starched and dressed his shirts, made him chest-protectors, muffettees, smoking-caps, neckcloths, purses, tobacco-pouches, slippers, braces' (Jane 1876).

This lengthy list of female labour brings to startling clarity the industry and planning required to realise the reified angel in the house.

Likewise, another anonymous female author debated woman's supposed inferiority in 'An Essay on the Moral Superiority of the Female Sex.' The author begins by emphasising the Christian virtue of the 'voluntary and graceful subordination of the wife to the husband' and assures the reader that the 'different organisations' of men and women fit them to 'different spheres of action' (An Essay on the Moral Superiority of the Female Sex 1879). However, despite these initially conservative arguments, the author insists on women's equality with men: 'it is denied that there is any natural inferiority in any of the qualities that distinguish the human race from the lower animals' (An Essay on the Moral Superiority of the Female Sex 1879). The nineteenth-century woman's evident weaknesses, the author suggests, might simply be a product of her environment. 'Hitherto the female sex has been inferior in the development of intellect' but 'the question is—comes the inferiority from nature or from bad education? Is it of Heaven or of men?' (An Essay on the Moral Superiority of the Female Sex 1879). The author argues that men's abuse of their 'superior physical strength' has deprived 'women of the means to evolve their capacities,' but in nations where 'the nearest approach to an equal education has been made [...] all authorities seem to say that girls do as well as the boys' (An Essay on the Moral Superiority of the Female Sex 1879). In a similar fashion to the female correspondents who replied to Maudsley, women at the CRI held on to preconceived notions about their role in society, at the same time as they challenged assumptions about women's intellectual capacities.

The informed debate in which female patients engaged in the pages of the *New Moon* was testament to their mental capabilities, both as women and as patients. Their journalistic contributions to the periodical demonstrate their interest in key political and cultural events occurring outside of the asylum. Crichton Royal kept a library which patients could access, with up-to-date journals and magazines (Turner 2019). Encouraged to maintain reading habits as part of the asylum's moral management therapeutics, female patients were able to remain knowledgeable about current affairs, including contemporary discussions over women's rights in titles such as the *Fortnightly Review*. The *New Moon* allowed female patients to express this knowledge and critically engage with social debates in a public forum. Publishing in the *New Moon* meant that their views would be heard by those in their circle (Crichton Royal's patient and staff population) and likely by a readership beyond the asylum walls. The publication thus gave the ideas of mentally ill, institutionalised women epistemological value and social capital. This contrasts strongly with the perception of patients given by the CRI case notes.

Amongst the female patients who weighed in on the discussion were Lydia Cairns and Helen S. Traill, two women who wrote vociferously for the *New Moon* during their time at the CRI. Lydia and Helen were two of the most frequent contributors to the periodical in the late 1870s, publishing a total of 12 and 20 contributions respectively. Both were middle-aged, single gentlewomen diagnosed with chronic mania, who appear to have caused considerable frustration in their caregivers.

Lydia Cairns was admitted, at age 45, in February 1862. Described as suffering from delusions that she is the Devil and has 'the power to possess them [others] with satanic powers,' her case is 'a most distressing one, almost an uninterrupted course of mental pain of the most acute kind' (CRI Case Book Vol. 12 1859–1864). During her first months in the asylum, she became increasingly anxious to leave, irritating her attendants by trying to get away 'incessantly' and being constantly 'on the lookout' for opportunities to escape (CRI Case Book Vol. 12 1859–1864). Her physician also describes her as exasperatingly narcissistic in her thoughts: 'the most trivial circumstances she fancies are especially designed to indicate something to her' (CRI Case Book Vol. 12 1859–1864). With 'no improvement in the case' after 7 years, Lydia was 'discharged on probation' in 1869, only to be readmitted in 1874 (CRI Case Book Vol. Vol. 14 1870–1876). The case notes from this later period state that she must be 'kept strictly in hand' (CRI Case Book Vol. 14 1870–1876). The physician writes with cruel humour that 'she still believes that she is a fiend or something the like one. She evidently is not far wrong if noise, distraction, and an obscene' manner are anything to be judged by (CRI Case Book Vol. 14 1870–1876).

Similarly, Helen S. Traill, admitted in June 1874 at 41, is described as 'one of our most troublesome patients' (CRI Case Book Vol. 14 1870–1876). She is 'always asking favours' and 'teasing everyone' (CRI Case Book Vol. 14. 1870–1876). Significantly, Helen's bad behaviour appears to be the predominant feature of her disorder; the notes state that 'beyond her excitability' and 'sham sentimentalism' there is 'no marked feature of insanity in her case' (CRI Case Book Vol. 14. 1870–1876). She is intensely disliked by her caregivers and thought to be 'irritable and nasty' (CRI Case Book Vol. 14. 1870–1876). Her physician is most annoyed with her demanding and selfish behaviour: 'her wants are so numerous that she has to be denied' (CRI Case Book Vol. 14. 1870–1876). In 1875, Helen was discharged and readmitted as a voluntary patient, presumably because her lack of symptoms made continued certification impossible. However, the physician remarks grumpily that 'it is exceedingly evident that the liberty accorded to this lady has been misdirected and misapplied,' for 'she is far more difficult to manage' (CRI Case Book Vol. 14. 1870–1876).

The case notes for both women evidence a lack of respect for the patients on the part of the medical assistants and, in a similar manner to the cases described above, suggest that Crichton Royal's doctors found their behaviour offensive. Lydia and Helen experienced periods of extreme psychological distress whilst at the asylum. However, most of their caregivers perceived this distress as disobedient and unreasonable. As unmarried women past their childbearing years, they may have induced subconscious prejudices in the men treating them; feelings which were likely compounded by the women's loud and demanding behaviour. Nevertheless, Lydia and Helen's thoughtful and engaged contributions to the *New Moon* are strikingly different to the picture of unreason painted by the case notes. Although the periodical was viewed by asylum staff as a civilising therapy, it was also a space in which patients were taken seriously as rational human beings. In the case notes, Lydia and Helen are dismissed, but publishing in the *New Moon* ensured that their ideas were recognised and valued.

Lydia published an article titled 'Woman's Suffrage' (Cairns 1877–1878), which appeared between December 1877 and January 1878. Votes for women was a subject then under discussion in the wider press. Single women ratepayers had gained the right to vote in local elections through the Municipal Franchise Act of 1869 and the male franchise had been extended in 1867. The question of female political responsibility was hotly debated as women began to enter higher education and the professions. Lydia had been gifted a copy of *The Woman's Suffrage Journal* whilst at Crichton Royal (presumably from another patient or staff member) and was requested to write about its contents in the *New Moon*. It thus appears that she was a known expert on the topic, or at least a recognised intellect within her community, who was eager to hear her views. Her article is a nuanced and attentive handling of the question, demonstrating a considerable amount of reasoning power.

Lydia initially presents women's suffrage as inevitable. The time has already come, she says, 'when women talkers are supposed to be women thinkers, and women's suffrage will be yielded' (Cairns 1877–1878). She suggests that many men would be 'right glad to let women do as they ask, fight their own battles' (Cairns 1877–1878). Indeed, she acknowledges that there are many classes of men who are not worthy of public office and who are 'conscious of their own mental weakness' (Cairns 1877–1878). However, Lydia does not write in support of votes for women. She argues that, whilst women might be capable of winning suffrage, it does not follow that they *should* do so. Woman 'should not ask for political responsibility, not because she is man's inferior, but because the range of her influence is higher than his' (Cairns 1877–1878). Women have an innate sense of morality, a God-given 'sense of right,' which makes their true home outside of the public eye: 'has not woman another sphere to occupy—the influence of the home—the first and earliest and deepest influences on the future statesmen and the future and present voters?' (Cairns 1877–1878). Women must 'exercise this power for good,' by instilling these values into future generations (Cairns 1877–1878).

Here Lydia sets up her political position, which is based on the essentialist belief that women are naturally virtuous. She then justifies this position, arguing her case with political acumen by raising potential counterarguments and dealing with them in turn. First, she argues that altering woman's sphere of action risks decreasing the moral power she holds over the family through the 'exciting and destructive influence of life's inevitable context' (Cairns 1877–1878). Next, Lydia acknowledges that 'it may be objected that the writer is combating a state of things which is not anticipated—that suffrage is not asked for any woman who is represented by the head of the household in which she finds her home' (Cairns 1877–1878). To this, she says that 'all political changes involve a change of principle'; in this case, 'it gives to women political power' (Cairns 1877–1878). Again, this is a power which women are not naturally designed to hold. Lydia also reminds the reader that political power is based on a principle of 'property qualification,' which under the present plans would see most female voters 'to be very young, or very old, or widows, whose every thought and energy is needed to obtain the daily bread of their fatherless children' (Cairns 1877–1878). She presents a logical case for women to refuse suffrage: political power would damage women's natural sphere of influence, and the proposed franchise (which makes concessions to this idea) is not based on sound principle. In fact, she argues that gaining the vote would not achieve the social change supporters desire: 'it appears to the writer that the question as to women's social rights is quite distinct from her asking for political power to obtain them' (Cairns 1877–1878).

Lydia displays advanced critical thinking skills which belie the mental disorder described in her case notes. 'Woman's Suffrage' not only highlights her capacity for reason (which was the periodical's therapeutic purpose) but is evidence of Lydia's existing ability to engage intellectually. Her article demonstrates considerable political awareness and detailed knowledge about the debate. She recalls arguments by previous campaigners, knows statistics about the population of women supposed to be represented by the vote, and understands where political responsibility lies in each case. To write such an engaged response, she must have been regularly reading and reflecting on the discussion in the press. Lydia was able to comprehend the content she read and form an informed opinion on a complex social issue. Yet this information is missing from Lydia's case notes which, as a clinical record, are narrowly focused on her symptoms of insanity and include little about her thoughts or interests. There is a diminished sense of personhood in these records which is restored in the non-clinical space of the periodical.

The *New Moon*'s therapeutic ideology of reason through refinement gave the periodical a cultural and intellectual focus and encouraged patients to express their beliefs and ideas. Turner (2019) and Daskalova (2022) have both observed that the *New Moon* and other asylum periodicals aimed to mimic highbrow titles on the mainstream market to assert their 'own value' and 'contributors' worth as thinking, rational subjects' (Daskalova 2022, p. 22). Turner has argued that the *New Moon* replicated the style of literary periodicals such as the quarterlies and literary annuals of the 1820s and 30s (Turner 2019, p. 78). She suggests that the magazine enacted the 'ideological tendencies, structures, forms, content, and thematic emphasis' of these periodicals as 'identifying features of "external" culture,' which 'lent the house organ a particular credibility' (Turner 2019, p. 81). Styling itself as a literary monthly, the *New Moon* regularly published discursive essays, where the author gave their opinion on topical subjects. This style of article was common within the quarterly reviews and, later in the century, within monthly magazines such as the *Fortnightly Review* and *Macmillan's Magazine* (Turner 2000; Worth 2003; Brake 2006; Shattock 2009; Finkelstein 2015). The literary quality of the periodical, and the discursive writing it encouraged, enabled Lydia to give voice to her ideas.

The opportunity to express herself in this fashion appears to have provided Lydia significant relief from her mental symptoms. Lydia was a long-term patient at the CRI, resident at the asylum for a total of 13 years, broken by a spell at Murray's Asylum in Perth. During this time, she experienced persistent, debilitating delusions and emotional insanity. The medical assistant noted, after her return from Perth in 1875, that her symptoms had 'not diminished in quantity or quality' (CRI Case Book Vol. 14 1870–1875). However, Lydia did not begin writing for the *New Moon* until 1876, her first contribution appearing in August of that year. It was then that there was a marked and sudden change in her behaviour. In May 1876, the medical assistant wrote that she is 'quarrelsome, irritable and impudent to officers and attendants. She believes she is the devil' (CRI Case Book Vol. 14 1870–1875). Yet, in December (7 months later and a mere 4 months after her first article was published) the case notes state that she 'is very industrious and makes many nice things' (CRI Case Book Vol. 14 1870–1875). She is 'sometimes a little noisy but always seems good natured' (CRI Case Book Vol. 14 1870–1875). Her delusions also began to wane, and the physician recorded in 1877 that 'Miss Cairns has for six months past behaved very well' (CRI Case Book Vol. 14 1870–1875). Lydia remained in good mental health and was discharged in July 1880.

Between 1876 and her discharge, Lydia regularly wrote for the *New Moon*, submitting approximately 3 contributions a year with a mix of topical articles and poetry. There is therefore a strong correlation between her literary activities and the alleviation of her mental illness. Writing appears to have significantly decreased her distress, which the case notes indicate she felt intensely: '[she] cries out that she is a painful unworthy creature and will never get better and return home' (CRI Case Book Vol. 12 1859–1864). For Lydia, the *New Moon* was a successful therapeutic instrument as it allowed her to exercise her intellectual faculties. Although the therapy was designed to teach patients reason, it also provided a welcome means of expression for those whose lively intelligence was suppressed by institutional life. The medical assistant admitted that Lydia possessed 'reasoning powers and knowledge' and that 'she can converse sensibly on many subjects,' often being 'very philosophical' in conversation (CRI Case Book Vol. 12 1859–1864). However, these traits were overshadowed, in the clinical setting of the asylum, by Lydia's 'exceedingly bad' behaviour (CRI Case Book Vol. 14 1870–1875). The medical assistant also dismissed her attempts to converse, finding her 'obtuse' (CRI Case Book Vol. 14 1870–1875). In contrast, the *New Moon* was a space in which Lydia could give full reign to her 'reasoning powers,' sharing her opinions with a grateful readership. The periodical offered Lydia personal expression, communication with her peers, and relieved the boredom of institutionalisation by providing much needed mental stimulation. From the perspective of asylum staff, the periodical also served its purpose in regulating Lydia's behaviour.

The writing of Helen S. Traill further demonstrates how patients' submissions to the *New Moon* could be personally fulfilling whilst also meeting asylum expectations. Helen was one of the earliest patients to discuss the woman question in the *New Moon*. In her article titled 'A Lady', published in the July 1875 number of the magazine, Helen endeavoured 'to pourtray [sic], in a few words, the lineaments of a "Lady"' (Traill 1875). The capitalisation of the noun reveals that the woman discussed here is an idealised figure; that ubiquitous Victorian archetype which linked virtue to both gender and social status. In her article, Helen defines an ideal of femininity which combines conservative, Christian values with a class-based ideology. Similarly to Lydia, Helen emphasises the inherent virtue of women. She describes how 'a Lady's duties are centred in her home, and within this hallowed enclosure the full and beauteaous play of her endearing qualities is seen to the greatest advantage' (Traill 1875). Through her essentially feminine attributes of kindness and selflessness, the Lady thinks always of the 'comfort, convenience, and interests of those associated with her, and finds the highest enjoyment in promoting their happiness' (Traill 1875). She is the ministering angel who supports 'the whole domestic edifice in every Christian household' (Traill 1875). The Lady's domestic duties are her 'divinely appointed privileges,' ordained by God (Traill 1875).

Helen's arguments are based in a Christian value system which saw the family as the source of moral wellbeing within society (Ginzberg 1990; Gleadle 2001; Griffin 2012). This value system relied on a class-specific domestic environment that allowed for women to be outside of the economic system whilst still providing for the wants of the family. Helen is explicit about the social status of her ideal Lady. The perfect woman has three roles: she is a 'wife, a mother, and a mistress' (Traill 1875). Sustaining these 'holy relationships' is crucial, as it is through them that the Lady exerts her moral influence (Traill 1875). In 'every relation of life' she is 'a friend and adviser to her husband, to her children, and to her servants' (Traill 1875). Helen thus emphasises women's domestic role in society through the reification of the upper-middle-class Lady as the moral and spiritual guardian of the family and nation. It is her natural (and it is implied, well-bred) purity and delicacy that allows her to guide others; 'refinement, cheerfulness, good-temper, true feeling and sympathy, and the ornament of a meek and quiet spirit, are the characteristics of a Christian Lady' (Traill 1875). Such women are the '"polished corners of the Temple"' (Traill 1875).

The character of the ideal woman which Helen describes is in direct contrast to the behaviour she exhibits in the asylum. She has a 'nasty' attitude, cares most for herself above all others, and 'behaves in a very emotional manner' (CRI Case Book Vol. 15 1870–1875). Helen's insanity is chiefly characterised by actions which are the opposite of those expected of a Lady. Yet her article is well reasoned, carefully written, and demonstrative of the civilised refinement praised within. It is possible to read Helen's article as evidence of the *New Moon*'s success as a therapeutic instrument. In writing 'A Lady', Helen has clearly reflected on appropriate ladylike behaviour and she appears to endorse values which bear significantly on her own case. As Turner has argued, it was the asylum's objective, through the 'reading and writing activities' provided, 'to enable patients to understand, reflect, and enact the societal norms of "civil", "outside" culture' (Turner 2019, p. 4). A 'heightened civility' was correlated with 'developed sanity' (Turner 2019, p. 38). Jill McMillan has even suggested that 'the magazine [...] forced contributors to internalise rational or sane thinking' (McMillan 2008, p. 50). Helen's class-specific vision of feminine good behaviour is reflective of the 'civilised' attitude encouraged at the CRI and is an aspirational model appropriate to the social station of the asylum's paying patients. Her article can therefore be considered in part a product of Crichton Royal's moral management ethos.

However, deeper investigation suggests that writing for the *New Moon* provided Helen with considerable personal satisfaction and was not merely a clinical exercise set by asylum staff. Helen's case notes reveal that one of the recurring features of her disorder was a 'mania for writing letters' (CRI Case Book Vol. 15 1870–1875). This behaviour continued throughout her stay at Crichton Royal, the medical assistant stating in March 1875 that 'her passion for writing letters has not subsided,' and again four months later, 'her writing propensity has not subsided' (CRI Case Book Vol. 15 1870–1875). Such enthusiastic letter writing implies that Helen had an unmet need for mental stimulation and personal expression, which the asylum periodical might provide. It is possible that staff recognised this need and indicated the *New Moon* as an appropriate employment for her, but there is no record of this, and she may have become involved with the periodical of her own volition. In any case, Helen took full advantage of the opportunity and began publishing her writing shortly after her arrival, with her first contribution appearing in August 1874. Helen published frequently, with at least one of her works appearing in the periodical every month between March and November 1875. She wrote travelogues, an article on gardening, and numerous poems, many of which expressed her sincere Christian faith. The contributions also continued after she left the asylum in 1876, with 3 submissions appearing between November 1878 and January 1879. As an ex-patient Helen may have continued to subscribe to the *New Moon* and it is likely that she sent in contributions from outside the institution. This suggests that Helen found genuine enjoyment in participating in the periodical. It was an activity in which she enthusiastically and voluntarily engaged.

The *New Moon* can therefore also be understood as a valuable intellectual and creative outlet for a woman whose strong desire to write was otherwise pathologised. Helen's article illustrates that patients' periodical writing was the result of both institutional influences and personal motivation. These complexities are highlighted by the contradictions inherent in 'A Lady'. Helen's act of writing for the *New Moon* undermined the conservative values she espoused. Journalistic work was a public, professional activity more akin to the rights demanded by reformers than the domestic feminine ideal which Helen endorsed. Yet public discussion was fundamental to the therapeutics of the *New Moon*, which was intended not only to encourage but to showcase intellectual refinement and serve as a positive example of mental health. In the context of the asylum periodical, Helen's desire to express her political and social opinions was perceived as respectable and she saw no contradiction between her conservative beliefs and writing for the *New Moon*. However, Helen's noisy behaviour elsewhere in the asylum was frowned upon and the medical assistants tried to encourage quietness, meekness, and industry; all attributes praised in 'A Lady.'

Despite these complexities, the *New Moon* was a space in which both Lydia and Helen could express their individuality and engage in intellectual debate. This opportunity was extended to patients of both sexes and women were valued thinkers and contributors to the magazine. Such a space was only possible due to Crichton Royal's moral management methodology, which encouraged patients to develop their reason through mental occupation, regardless of gender. The periodical writing of female patients at the CRI must therefore be considered within the wider context of the institution. The *New Moon* was a therapy designed to improve irrational behaviour and patients' writing was shaped by this ideology. Nevertheless, women's contributions to the *New Moon* demonstrate that female asylum patients were not merely the oppressed victims which previous historiography has suggested. In enabling women to engage creatively and critically in public debate, the periodical offered Lydia and Helen greater representation than they achieved in their daily lives outside the asylum.

Conclusion

The written record of the asylum reveals that there was considerable variation and nuance in the experiences of female patients at the Crichton Royal Institution. The casebooks show that women were treated with a degree of contempt on the ward, depending on how well their behaviour met staff expectations. Yet, in the asylum periodical which was such an important part of life at Crichton Royal, women were given agency and respect and found enjoyment in their work. Such records are evidence of women's experiences at the asylum, but they also played a role in shaping them. Classificatory tools like the Register of Lunatics and occupational therapies such as the *New Moon* were instruments through which the institution implemented its clinical methodologies and directly impacted patients' lives.

Crucially, these texts demonstrate that the clinical approach at the CRI was driven primarily by moral management principles, rather than ideologies of gender. Under a system in which the cultivation of reason was of primary importance to the cure of insanity, factors such as patients' sex became a secondary consideration. The experiences of female patients at the CRI were only partially shaped by doctors' beliefs about women, or psychiatric theories specific to the female mind. Reading asylum records and publications alongside other psychiatric literature is therefore vital to developing a full understanding of nineteenth-century attitudes to mentally ill women. Such records do not contradict the importance given, in medical textbooks, to the influence of female reproductive biology on the mind but rather provide evidence that the treatment of female insanity was often complex and involving multiple, sometimes competing, belief systems.

Crichton Royal Institution's treatment of its female patients in the 1870s and 1880s was the result of the institution's particular clinical methodology, its requirement to provide a comfortable standard of care for paying patients, and the wider context of the professionalisation and increasing state regulation of psychiatry in Scotland after 1857. This unique blend of contextual factors was specific to the CRI. As scholarship has shown, other asylums around Britain faced different (if similar) contexts. In part, this was due to the continuing professionalisation of the discipline during the second half of the nineteenth century and the variety of institutional profiles which existed across the nation, from state-run pauper facilities to charitable institutions, and private houses. There was considerable variation in practice even at this period, which led to the uneven application of psychiatric theories even as they gained consensus in the profession. Shifting professional norms and developing disciplinary methodologies were thus as influential as social ideologies in shaping psychiatric theories about the female brain.

References

Unpublished Sources

Crichton Royal Institution Case Book Vol. 12. 1859–1864. Wellcome Collection. DGH1/5/21/1/12.

Crichton Royal Institution Case Book Vol. 14. 1870–1876. Wellcome Collection. DGH1/5/21/1/14.

Crichton Royal Institution Case Book, Vol. 15. 1876–1881. Wellcome Collection. DGH1/5/21/1/15.

Crichton Royal Institution Case Book, Vol. 16. 1881–1885. Wellcome Collection. DGH1/5/21/1/16.

Crichton Royal Institution Register of Lunatics. 1839–1878. Wellcome Collection. DGH1/5/2/1.

Crichton Royal Institution Register of Lunatics. 1878–1884. Wellcome Collection. DGH1/5/2/2.

Crichton Royal Institution Sherrif's Warrants. 1838–1936. Wellcome Collection. DGH1/5/1/1.

Daskalova, Mila. 2022. Printing and Periodical Culture in the Nineteenth-Century Asylum. PhD thesis: University of Strathclyde. https://doi.org/10.48730/js8s-vx55

Glenn Tinnin, Jonathan. 2019. Madness Narratives: Victorian Textual Responses to the Insanity Diagnosis. PhD thesis: University of Kentucky. https://doi.org/10.13023/etd.2019.441

Halliday, Emma Catherine. 2003. Themes in Scottish Asylum Culture. The Hospitalisation of the Scottish Asylum, 1880–1914. PhD thesis: University of Stirling. http://hdl.handle.net/1893/3265. Accessed 1 January 2025.

Jardine, Alex. 1880. *General Rules of the Crichton Royal Institution, Dumfries.* Wellcome Collection. DGH1/2/5/2.

McMillan, Jill. 2008. 'Writer Heal Thyself': The *New Moon,* Patient Agency and the Crichton Royal Institution. MA thesis: University of Guelph. https://hdl.handle.net/10214/20981. Accessed 1 January 2025.

NB: Print copies of the *New Moon; or, Crichton Royal Institution Literary Register* have been digitised and made available via the Wellcome Collection. DGH1/7/1/1.

Rice, Francis J. 1981. Madness and Industrial Society: A Study of the Origins and Early Growth of the Organisation of Insanity in Nineteenth-Century Scotland. PhD thesis: University of Strathclyde. https://doi.org/10.48730/rdv5-1v91

Turner, Emily Jessica. 2019. Patients' Creative Work and 'Expressive Possibilities' in *New Moon*, *Under the Dome*, and the *Hydra*, 1844–1918. PhD thesis: University of Sussex. https://hdl.handle.net/10779/uos.23475773.v1. Accessed 1 January 2025.

Published Sources

A.C.M. 1876 (June). A Night in the House of Commons. *New Moon; or, Crichton Royal Institution Literary Register*. 32.

A Day at Giron. 1880 (March-May). *New Moon; or, Crichton Royal Institution Literary Register*. 36.

Allen Campbell, Morag. 2017. 'Noisy, Restless, and Incoherent': Puerperal Insanity at Dundee Lunatic Asylum. *History of Psychiatry*. 28: 44-57. https://doi.org/10.1177/0957154X16671262

Amusements, &c, During the Past Month. 1875 (December). *New Moon; or, Crichton Royal Institution Literary Register*. 31.

Andrews, Jonathan. 1997. A Failure to Flourish? David Yellowlees and the Glasgow School of Psychiatry: Part 2. *History of Psychiatry*. 8: 333–360. https://doi.org/10.1177/0957154X9700803102.

Andrews, Jonathan. 1998. Documents and Sources: Case Notes, Case Histories, and the Patient's Experience of Insanity at Gartnavel Royal Asylum, Glasgow, in the Nineteenth Century. *Social History of Medicine* 11: 255–281. https://doi.org/10.1093/shm/11.2.255.

An Essay on the Moral Superiority of the Female Sex. 1879 (July-August). *New Moon; or, Crichton Royal Institution Literary Register*, 35.

Barfoot, Michael, and Allan Beveridge. 1990. Madness at the Crossroads: John Home's Letters from the Royal Edinburgh Asylum, 1886–87. *Psychological Medicine*. 20: 263–284. https://doi.org/10.1017/s0033291700017591.

Barfoot, Michael, and Allan Beveridge. 1993. 'Our Most Notable Inmate': John Willis Mason at the Royal Edinburgh Asylum, 1864–1901. *History of Psychiatry*. 4: 159–208. https://doi.org/10.1177/0957154X9300401402.

Barret-Ducrocq, Françoise. 1991. *Love in the Time of Victoria: Sexuality, Class, and Gender in Nineteenth-Century London*, trans by. John Howe. London: Virago.

Beveridge, Allan. 1998. Life in the Asylum: Patients' Letters from Morningside, 1873–1908. *History of Psychiatry*. 9: 431–469. https://doi.org/10.1177/0957154X9800903602.

Brake, Laurel. Maga, the Shilling Monthlies, and the New Journalism. In *Print Culture and the Blackwood Tradition, 1805–1930*, ed. by David Finkelstein, 184–211. Toronto: University of Toronto Press.

Browne, W.A.F. 1837. *What Asylums Were, Are, and Ought to Be: Being the Substance of Five Lectures Delivered Before the Managers of the Montrose Royal Lunatic Asylum.* Edinburgh: Adam and Charles Black.

Cairns, Lydia. 1877 (December)-1878 (January). Woman's Suffrage. *New Moon; or, Crichton Royal Institution Literary Register*, 33.

Chaney, Sarah. 2015. Useful Members of Society or Motiveless Malingerers? Occupation and Malingering in British Asylum Psychiatry. In *Waltraud Ernst, 277–297*, ed. Psychiatry Work and Society, c.1750–2015, 1870–1914. Manchester: Manchester University Press.

Chaney, Sarah. 2016. 'No 'Sane' Person Would Have Any Idea': Patients' Involvement in Late Nineteenth-Century British Asylum Psychiatry. *Medical History.* 60: 37–53. https://doi.org/10.1017/mdh.2015.67

Charland, Louis C. 2007. Benevolent Theory: Moral Treatment at the York Retreat. *History of Psychiatry.* 18: 61–80. https://doi.org/10.1177/0957154X07070320.

Charland, Louis C. 2012. Benevolence and Discipline: The Concept of Recovery in Early Nineteenth-Century Moral Treatment. In *Recovery of People with Mental Illness: Philosophical and Related Perspectives*, ed. Abraham Rudnick, 64–77. Oxford: Oxford University Press.

Cromhall Easterbrook, Charles. 1937. *The Chronicle of Crichton Royal.* Dumfries: Courier Press.

Daskalova, Mila. 2021. Printing as Poison, Printing as Cure: Work and Health in the Nineteenth-Century Printing Office and Asylum. *Book History.* 24: 58–84. https://doi.org/10.1353/bh.2021.0002.

de Young, Mary. 2015. *Encyclopedia of Asylum Therapeutics, 1750–1950.* Jefferson: McFarland & Company.

Digby, Anne. 1985. *Madness, Morality and Medicine: A Study of the York Retreat, 1796–1914.* Cambridge: Cambridge University Press.

Ellis, Robert, Sarah Kendal, and Steven J. Taylor, eds. 2021. *Voices in the History of Madness: Personal and Professional Perspectives on Mental Health and Illness.* Cham: Palgrave Macmillan.

Erlana. 1876 (April-July). A Projected Tour of the West of Ireland. *New Moon; or, Crichton Royal Institution Literary Register*, 32.

Finkelstein, David. 2015. The Role of the Literary and Cultural Periodical. In *The Routledge Companion to British Media History*, ed. Martin Conboy and John Steel, 263–272. Abingdon: Routledge.

F.M. 1876 (April-June). Colour. *New Moon; or, Crichton Royal Institution Literary Register*, 32.

Ginzberg, Lori D. 1990. *Women and the Work of Benevolence: Morality, Politics and Class in the Nineteenth-Century United States*. New Haven: Yale University Press.

Gleadle, Kathryn. 2001. *British Women in the Nineteenth Century*. Basingstoke: Palgrave.

Gorham, Deborah. 1982. *The Victorian Girl and the Feminine Ideal*. London: Routledge.

Griffin, Ben. 2012. *The Politics of Gender in Victorian Britain: Masculinity, Political Culture and the Struggle for Women's Rights*. Cambridge: Cambridge University Press.

Hanganu-Bresch, Cristina, and Carol Berkenkotter. 2012. Narrative Survival: Personal and Institutional Accounts of Asylum Confinement. *Literature and Medicine*. 30: 12–41. https://doi.org/10.1353/lm.2012.0006.

Hill, Simon A., and Richard Laugharne. 2003. Mania, Dementia and Melancholia in the 1870s: Admissions to a Cornwall Asylum. *Journal of the Royal Society of Medicine*. 96: 361–363. https://doi.org/10.1177/014107680309600719.

Holligan, Christopher. 2024. Educative Psychological Treatment at Edinburgh's Royal Asylum: Unfolding *The Morningside Mirror*, 1845–1882. *Social History of Medicine*. https://doi.org/10.1093/shm/hkae022.

In Memoriam D.F. 1875 (February). *New Moon; or, Crichton Royal Institution Literary Register*, 31.

Jane, Hilda Evelyn. 1876 (May-September). Lecture: Ladies, Would-Be's [sic] and Women. *New Moon; or, Crichton Royal Institution Literary Register*. 32.

Lazenby Craig, Barbara. 1989. Hospital Records and Record-Keeping, C. 1850-C. 1950, Part I: The Development of Records in Hospitals. *Archivaria,* 29: 57-87.

Lazenby Craig, Barbara. 1991. The Role of Records and of Recordkeeping in the Development of the Modern Hospital in London, England, and Ontario, Canada, c.1890-1940. *Bulletin of the History of Medicine*. 65: 367-397.

Lydia. 1876 (August-September). On British Associationism. *New Moon; or, Crichton Royal Institution Literary Register.* 32.

Marland, Hilary. 2004. *Dangerous Motherhood: Insanity and Childbirth in Victorian Britain*. Basingstoke: Palgrave Macmillan.

Mendus, Susan, and Jane Rendall. 1989. *Sexuality and Subordination: Interdisciplinary Studies of Gender in the Nineteenth Century*. London: Routledge.

Morrison, Hazel. 2013. Conversing with the Psychiatrist: Patient Narratives within Glasgow's Royal Asylum, 1921–1929. *Journal of Literature and Science*. 6: 18–37. https://doi.org/10.12929/jls.06.1.02

Morrison, Hazel. 2016. Constructing Patient Stories: 'Dynamic' Case Notes and Clinical Encounters at Glasgow's Gartnavel Mental Hospital, 1921–32. *Medical* History. 60: 67–86. https://doi.org/ https://doi.org/10.1017/mdh.2015.69

Newman, Sara. 2011. Disability and Life Writing: Reports from the Nineteenth Century Asylum. *Journal of Literary & Cultural Disability Studies.* 5: 261–278. https://doi.org/10.3828/jlcds.2011.22.

Our Christmas Tree for 1874. 1875 (January). *New Moon; or, Crichton Royal Institution Literary Register*, 31.

Philo, Chris, and Jonathan Andrews. 2017. Introduction: Histories of Asylums, Insanity and Psychiatry in Scotland. *History of Psychiatry.* 28: 3–14. https://doi.org/10.1177/0957154X16678566.

Porter, Roy. 1985. The Patient's View, Doing Medical History from Below. *Theory and Society.* 14: 175–198.

Risse, Guenter B., and Harley Warner. 1992. Reconstructing Clinical Activities: Patient Records in Medical History. *Social History of Medicine.* 5: 183–205. https://doi.org/10.1093/shm/5.2.183.

Savage, George Henry. 1884. *Insanity and Allied Neuroses: Practical and Clinical.* London: Cassell & Co.

Scottish Lunacy Commission. 1857. *Report by her Majesty's Commissioners appointed to inquire into the state of lunatic asylums in Scotland: and the existing law in reference to lunatics and lunatic asylums in that part of the United Kingdom.* Edinburgh: Thomas Constable.

Scull, Andrew. 2011. The Peculiarities of the Scots? Scottish Influence on the Development of English Psychiatry, 1700–1980. *History of Psychiatry.* 22: 403–415. https://doi.org/10.1177/0957154X10390496.

Scrine, Claire. 2003. Female Excess in the Age of Restraint: Conceptions of Nymphomania in Nineteenth-Century Medicine. *Lilith: A Feminist History Journal.* 12: 110–122.

Shattock, Joanne. 2009. Monthly Magazines. In *Dictionary of Nineteenth-Century Journalism in Great Britain and Ireland*, ed. by Laurel Brake and Marysa Demoor, 423. Ghent: Academia Press.

Skae, David. 1863. *Of the Classification of the Various Forms of Insanity on a Rational and Practical Basis: Being an Address Delivered at the Royal College of Physicians, London, at the Annual Meeting of the Association of Medical Officers of Asylums, on 9th July 1863.* Unidentified publisher.

Skultans, Veida. 1975. *Madness and Morals: Ideas on Insanity in the Nineteenth Century.* London: Routledge.

Smith Clouston, Thomas. 1893. The Lunacy Administration of Scotland, 1857-1892. *American Journal of Insanity.* 50: 186-197.

Traill, Helen S. 1875 (July). A Lady. *New Moon; or, Crichton Royal Institution Literary Register*, 31.

Turner, Mark W. 2000. *Trollope and the Magazines.* Basingstoke: Palgrave Macmillan.

Vicinus, Martha, ed. 1972. *Suffer and Be Still: Women in the Victorian Age.* London: Routledge.

Walsh, Lorraine. 2004. A Class Apart? Admissions to the Dundee Royal Lunatic Asylum, 1890–1910. In *Sex and Seclusion, Class and Custody: Perspectives on Gender and Class in the History of British and Irish Psychiatry*, ed. Jonathan Andrews and Anne Digby, 249–270. Amsterdam: Rodopi.

Worth, George J. 2003. *Macmillan's Magazine, 1859–1907: No Flippancy or Abuse Allowed*. Burlington: Ashgate.

CHAPTER 5

Making a Name for Herself: Helen Boyle's Work as a Female Pioneer in Mental Health Care

The preceding chapters have explored nineteenth-century theories and treatment of female insanity in depth. This book now moves beyond these discussions to examine how beliefs about the female mind impacted a different group of women involved with the psychiatric profession: those who worked within the field. As the response to Maudsley's 'Sex in Mind and in Education' has shown, women were fighting to join the British medical community from the 1870s, and over the following decades a significant minority of women were able to qualify as doctors and begin working. Psychiatry was one of the career pathways most open to them, in part because the stigma of asylum work meant that there was less competition for roles from male candidates. Several women secured jobs as mind doctors during the 1890s and were able to join the discipline's professional body, the Medio-Psychological Association (MPA), which had opened membership to female doctors in 1894. The final years of the nineteenth century were a pivotal moment in the history of women and psychiatry, as for the first time they had an influence on the medical treatment and theory of mental disease. This chapter will therefore begin in the last decade of the Victorian era before looking further, into the twentieth century, to investigate how female mind doctors faced the challenges of these early years, contending with gendered biases like those faced by female patients to become integrated into the profession. In doing so,

M. Chapman, *Writing Women's Madness, 1845–1914*, Palgrave Studies in Literature, Science and Medicine,
https://doi.org/10.1007/978-3-031-97092-4_5

this chapter will focus on one pioneering woman in particular: Dr Helen Boyle.

Helen Boyle was one of the first women to start working within an asylum in England and her career highlights the important role that sex and gender played in the progression of women within medicine. She enjoyed an extremely successful career, working at Claybury Asylum before opening her own institution in 1905, the Lady Chichester Hospital for nervous disorders, and eventually becoming the president of the MPA in 1939. Boyle's success was in large measure due to her ability to navigate the complexities of her position. As a female physician she was marginalised and the choices available to her, in entering the job market and selecting a field, were contingent on her sex. These restrictions fundamentally shaped the way in which Boyle could practise medicine, beginning from her early decision to take a job in mental health care. This chapter will follow Boyle's life and her ground-breaking work as a female doctor in mental disease, focusing on the time between her medical training in the early 1890s and the outbreak of World War 1 in 1914—an event which, aside from its global consequences, would spark significant changes to the practice of psychiatry in Britain. It will explore how Boyle's career was affected by contemporary beliefs about women's physical and mental capacities and how she was able to exploit a niche within psychiatry as a female mind doctor.

Boyle used an ideological strategy, which drew on various concepts of womanhood circulating at the turn of the century, to manage her professional and public image and argue for a rightful place within mind doctoring. This strategy encompassed both separatist and inclusionist tactics, which Boyle implemented to her advantage in different aspects of her career. These tactics are commonly utilised by individuals trying to break into a profession from which they have been excluded, either by forming a faction and operating in a novel manner to expand the discipline (separatism), or by assimilating themselves into the existing establishment (inclusionism). They are terms familiar within the historiography of the women's movement and are tactics which were employed by Boyle's female predecessors in medicine.

Mary Ann Elston (2001) has shown how the first women to enter the profession responded to opposition by arguing for the need for female doctors to treat female patients (and children). This was 'a strategy based on a complex mix of principle and pragmatism' and built on the claim that 'medical women had a specific mission to serve women's otherwise unmet health care needs' (Elston 2001, p. 77). Ideologically, such work was an extension of women's domestic and caring duties in the home. It also had the moral (and socially palatable) benefit of saving female patients the indignity of employing a male doctor for the delicate physical examinations which gynaecological or obstetric care might necessitate. Women doctors in the nineteenth century thus often pursued a policy of separatism, establishing their own hospitals solely for the treatment of women and children. Louise Westwood has described how separatism seemed to 'ensure a measure of clinical freedom' away from male supervision and the chance to fight against 'unequal pay, patriarchy and poor career opportunities' (Westwood 2006, p. 93). It also gave women a clear role in the medical marketplace through the separate treatment of female patients. Westwood has also shown that Boyle's 'founding of her own hospital [the Lady Chichester], using only women as consultants, was a separatist tactic' which followed in the footsteps of medical women before her (Westwood 2001, p. 456). In creating a 'network of female medical experts' Boyle avoided the difficulties faced by others of her sex, by 'stepp[ing] out of the competitive side of medicine' into a female-only 'working environment' (Westwood 2001, p. 456).

However, Boyle's approach to her professional life is more complex than what Westwood describes. Boyle followed two divergent paths in her clinical practice and in the management of her professional identity. In her clinical work Boyle took a separationist route as Westwood demonstrates, marking out discrete professional territory by arguing that female mental patients were best treated by a female physician. In this, Boyle recognised a gap in the medical marketplace and utilised the familiar concept of the medical woman's mandate to legitimise an unusual career choice: the establishment of the Lady Chichester Hospital (LCH) for the treatment of women in early mental illness. Despite this, Boyle also saw the benefits of being an active member of the mainstream alienist community. She was keen to join the MPA and regularly attended its quarterly meetings. Boyle used these inclusionist tactics to gather support amongst male colleagues for her innovative ideas and treatment practices. This support enabled her to build status for herself, consolidate her professional identity, and advance herself to positions of prestige in her career. Ultimately, Boyle was ambitious and made discrete choices at various points of her working life to progress as far as possible professionally, whether this was through gaining clinical freedom or promotion within the field. Understanding her biography in this way enables us to see how Boyle was motivated not just by the circumstances of her sex but by a tension between a desire for intellectual independence and the conventional markers of success.

Significantly, it was through her textual practices that Boyle was able to skilfully manipulate contemporary concepts of femininity and claim a place for herself within the medical profession. Boyle's story is therefore told through the texts which she, and the institutions she was part of, published. These texts enabled Boyle to communicate and tailor her vision for early treatment to different audiences. Using a two-pronged approach, Boyle first produced annual reports for the LCH which showcased her revolutionary work on early treatment of nervous disorders in women. These reports demonstrate her separatist theories in action, as Boyle drew on ideas of feminine domesticity and nurture to justify the unique role of her team of female physicians within the mind sciences. Secondly, Boyle gave papers at MPA meetings which were then published in the society's periodical, the *Journal of Mental Science*. Significantly, she did not utilise the same ideologies in these MPA papers as she did in her reports, where her womanhood was paramount. Instead, Boyle argued for the expansion of professionalisation within psychiatry to incorporate her field into mainstream practice.

Print was a tool which Boyle used to control her professional reputation, navigating the complexities of a career as a woman in mental health care at the end of the nineteenth century. Writing within different genres, she was able to construct narratives about herself and her work that helped her to lobby for what she wanted. She utilised the LCH annual reports to promote and defend aspects of her work which challenged established (male) practices in her field, whilst taking advantage of her MPA membership to give papers which built positive relationships with the mainstream of the profession. This chapter will examine Boyle's career and the texts she produced, placing her story within the wider context of women's entry into the medical professions.

Women in Late Nineteenth-Century Medicine and the Beginning of Boyle's Psychiatric Career

Alice Helen Anne Boyle was born in Dublin on 19th November 1869, into a middle-class family with a banker father (Milliken 2006, 2010).[1] At first educated at home, she later went to school in Bonn, Germany, where the family moved in 1882 after her father, Richard Boyle, became bankrupt. Boyle's parents later separated and in 1887 her mother, Alice, moved Helen and her siblings to England where her brothers continued to be schooled. By her late teens Boyle was in a position like many other girls of her class and situation in the late Victorian period. Decently educated, she was approaching maturity without the financial means for independence and needed to provide for herself through work or marriage. Boyle chose a career in medicine, a move which was supported by her family. A relation of her mother, Thomas K. Chambers, signed the testimonial for her admission to the London School of Medicine for Women (LSMW) in 1889, then the only institution in England open to girls wishing to receive medical training (Application Form 249: Helen Boyle 1889).[2] Boyle began classes in October of that year.

The London School of Medicine for Women

As discussed in Chapter 3, the LSMW was founded in October 1874 by Sophia Jex-Blake with the purpose of providing a medical education for women. The story of the school's foundation reflects the difficulties encountered by the professional women who paved the way for Boyle's generation (Elston 1986; Bourdillon 1988; Blake 1990; Thomson 1998; Hardy and Conrad 2001; Crowther and Dupree 2007; McIntyre 2014). The LSMW's original council included many key players in the medical and biological sciences, such as Elizabeth Garrett Anderson, John Hughlings Jackson and Thomas Huxley. Several council members, including Garrett Anderson, also taught on the curriculum. Lectures

[1] Helen Boyle's only biographer has been Emma Milliken, who wrote the Dictionary of National Biography entry on Boyle (2006), as well as a doctoral thesis on her life and medical career (2010). All details of Helen Boyle's biography have been taken from these sources, unless otherwise indicated.

[2] Thomas Chambers wrote that he had known Helen 'all her life' and '[I] think she will be a credit to the school.'

were held in a range of subjects such as anatomy, physiology, botany, materia medica, midwifery, surgery, and pathology, and took place at the LSMW's well-located premises on Brunswick Square in Bloomsbury, London (LSMW Prospectus 1874). The school grew quickly, adding new subjects to the curriculum and securing aristocratic patronage on the board (LSMW Prospectus 1875). Despite this promising start, however, there remained much resistance to female physicians from both the professional community and lay people.

One significant difficulty the school faced was finding clinical instruction for its students. This hands-on experience was a vital addition to the curriculum as it was necessary for them to qualify and practise as doctors. It was not until three years after the school's foundation that students at the LSMW could take clinical classes alongside their lectures, on the Royal Free Hospital's teaching programme (LSMW Prospectus 1877). In addition, when the LSMW opened women still had no right to attend any of the colleges which were certified to offer the qualifying exams in medicine. Again, the LSMW needed the support and cooperation of external institutions. Entry to the Boards was only achieved through a parliamentary Bill in 1876, which '"enabled" (without compelling) all British Examining Boards to extend their examinations and qualifications to women' (Jex-Blake 1887). At the same time 'the question was brought by the Government before the Medical Council' who said that they were '"not prepared to say that women ought to be excluded from the profession"' (Jex-Blake 1887). Although these changes meant that women were technically afforded access to all aspects of medical training by the late 1870s, the language of these reports demonstrates the lack of enthusiasm felt by the profession. The admittance of women to the Boards was still a choice left very much to each individual college (Witz 1992; McIntyre 2014).

During the following decade supporters continued to campaign for change and by the 1890s a complete medical education was at last available to both sexes. When Boyle entered the LSMW in 1889, the school offered the full theoretical and clinical medical curriculum and had also fostered links with examining bodies for its students to take their qualifications. Once students held their diplomas they could apply for a place on the Medical Register. The 1889–1890 prospectus lists 18 courses available to students, including ophthalmic surgery, diseases of women, forensic medicine and hygiene, and organic chemistry. Individuals could specialise in areas relevant to their career path or take a general route to qualify as a doctor. Hospital instruction comprised clinical lectures given fortnightly by each of the four senior members of the Royal Free staff, alternating between clinical surgery and clinical medicine. Demonstrations were held on auscultation and physical signs, ward work, surgery, pathology, pharmacy, and anaesthetics. Several certified universities and colleges across England, Scotland and Ireland now admitted women to their medical examinations. These included the University of London, the King and Queen's College of Physicians and the Royal College of Surgeons, Ireland, and the Royal College of Physicians and Royal College of Surgeons, Edinburgh (LSMW Prospectus 1889).

From the outset, Helen Boyle aimed to obtain an MD. On her admission form for the school, she declared her intention to 'pursue a complete course of qualifying medical study, and to present [herself] in due course to the Examining Boards with a view to obtaining a registrable diploma' (Application Form 349: Helen Boyle 1889). This ambition is reflected in the wide range of courses she chose during her studies. Variety appears to have suited Boyle, as she did well in many of her classes, coming 2nd in class in ordinary chemistry, 4th in anatomy in her first year and 1st in her second, 3rd in midwifery and gynaecology, and 7th in surgery. She also took materia medica, physiology, pathology, medicine, and operative midwifery (which, alas, did not seem to be her forte: she came bottom of class) (LSMW Results of School Examinations 1874–1900). She graduated from the LSMW in 1893, sitting the Scottish triple qualification in medicine and becoming a licentiate of the Royal College of Physicians and Royal College of Surgeons of Edinburgh. By 1894 she had sat for her MD in Brussels and joined the British Medical Association as a qualified doctor (C.L.H 1957).[3] She also began volunteering at Canning Town Medical Mission whilst looking for paid employment, working as a general practice physician caring for East London's poor. Boyle had thus fulfilled the goal she set out for herself on her admission form in 1889 and was already on track to establishing herself in clinical practice.

[3] European universities had long accepted women to the medical examinations and many female physicians chose to qualify abroad rather than in Britain. Brussels was a popular option because it was cheaper than other universities, a factor which motivated Boyle's choice.

Boyle's Entry into Psychiatry

However, only a few months later in January 1895, she took up the post of Fifth Assistant Medical Officer at the London County Council asylum, Claybury (Claybury Sub-Committee Minutes 1895–1896). This decision is surprising considering Boyle's career aspirations and experience. The LSMW did offer a course in mental pathology, which was initiated in 1875 and originally taught by W.H.O. Sankey (of textbook fame). During Boyle's tenure at the school the course was led by the renowned Charles Mercier and included 12 lectures on subjects such as the function of the nervous system, constitution of mind, and the nature and treatment of insanity (LSMW Prospectus 1875 and 1889). Yet mental pathology was not one of the many classes which Boyle attended; there is no record of Boyle on Mercier's class lists, or of her being examined in the subject (LSMW Results of School Examinations 1874–1900). The class in mental pathology was optional, not being a requirement for a medical diploma at the time, and Boyle's choice of subjects was clearly focused on those necessary for the qualifying examinations. Indeed, there is no indication that she was intending to specialise in mental health care. Her acceptance of the role at Claybury is therefore unlikely to have been motivated by her professional goals.

One explanation for such a move was the poor availability of work for women in medicine when Boyle graduated in the mid-1890s. Like many female doctors at the end of the nineteenth century, Boyle's prospects were limited, and her early career choices were likely dictated by the small range of options open to her at the time. Many medical roles, particularly those of higher status or greater specialisation, were simply not offered to women (Elston 1986). As Claire Brock has shown, a stigma still existed around employing female doctors due to their perceived 'inability to cope with the strains of the profession, their physical inferiority rendering them incapable of dealing with the "hard labour" involved in the practice of medicine' (Brock 2007). However, arguments based on traditional ideas of femininity, such as women's innate suitability for philanthropy or the need for a doctor to show modesty and discretion in treatment, meant that certain roles were easier to come by than others: in particular, jobs which involved the care of female patients (Elston 1986; Blake 1990).

In the 1890s, Claybury Asylum trialled a policy of hiring female physicians to work on their female wards. Opportunities for women medical officers were advertised at the time of Boyle's return from Brussels. She applied for the role and was interviewed by the Claybury sub-committee, who hired her on the spot, offering a salary of £120 per annum, with board, lodging and washing (Claybury Sub-Committee Minutes 1894–1895). This was equal pay to male medical officers at the asylum. In addition, although Claybury had only recently opened in 1893, it already had a reputation for its progressive approach to the treatment of insanity. Its superintendent, Robert Armstrong Jones, was young, skilled, and innovative (Hide 2014, p. 43). The London County Council had also approved the addition of a pathological laboratory and the appointment of leading neurophysiologist Frederick Mott as pathologist, who joined Claybury around the same time as Boyle, in 1895 (Buklijas 2017). It is probable that the job, specifically for a female doctor, on good pay, and at a new institution with a scientific focus, seemed to Boyle like a more appealing option than many of the other roles on the market. For once, her sex meant she was aptly suited to the position and made it more rather than less likely that she would be hired. Although she had no particular interest in psychiatry at the time, asylum work for women was more readily available than roles in disciplines less desperate for employees. These circumstances ultimately led to her future success as a female alienist, for whilst she may have stumbled into the field, the two years she spent at Claybury were to ignite in Boyle a life-long interest in mental health care.

At the asylum, Boyle undertook all the usual tasks required of an assistant medical officer. Louise Hide has described the 'formidable range of duties' expected of asylum officers, including 'overseeing admissions procedures, [...] dealing with disturbed patients,' and classifying patients 'according to behaviour and symptoms' (Hide 2014, p. 49). Added to this were 'the onerous demands of asylum bureaucracy' (Hide 2014, p. 49). Although the work was hard and the role junior, the intellectual environment was progressive and Boyle had the opportunity to work with Mott in his laboratory, where she excelled. In fact, during her investigations she became the first person to identify and isolate the bacillus for dysentery, an infectious condition common amongst mental patients (Milliken 2006).

On top of his interest in the microbial origins of mental disease, Mott was also concerned with the poor and ineffectual treatment of patients in the early stages of insanity. As Tatjana Buklijas has described, the London County Council's main motivation in setting up the pathological laboratory was to investigate 'the prevention of mental illness' and thus alleviate the heavy burden of patients dependent on asylum care (Buklijas 2017, p. 317). Mott believed that the onset of nervous disease was a crucial moment for intervention. Preventing the disease from progressing was vital to stop the patient ending up in permanent care. He later lobbied for 'Receiving Houses [...] as replacement hospitals for the acutely insane,' where patients could go during their first episode of illness instead of being sent to the asylum (Buklijas 2017, p. 317). This 'promised to cut costs and avoid the stigma attached to asylums, while at the same time providing the researcher with material to study the onset of mental illness' (Buklijas 2017, p. 317). Boyle therefore not only witnessed first-hand the problems of an over-full asylum and the delays in treatment this caused for her patients but worked closely with those who had reformist views about an alternative solution to long-term institutionalisation of the insane. This experience would stick with her and Boyle would later cite Mott as a key influence on her own thinking about early treatment (Boyle 1939).

However, although Claybury was intellectually significant for Boyle, professionally speaking there was very little scope for improvement. Hide has shown how despite Claybury's open-minded policies there were considerable frictions created by 'the disruption female doctors caused within a distinctly male working environment' (Hide 2014, p. 46). The women medical officers 'battled contempt and scorn that was liberally meted out by patients, nurses, and male colleagues alike'; male medical officers in particular 'resented the intrusion of women into their professional space, ostensibly on equal terms' (Hide 2014, p. 59). These tensions, coupled with the assault of some of the female medical staff by patients, meant that by 1901 the asylum made the decision to stop employing women doctors. Boyle had resigned from her post a few years earlier, in January 1897. We cannot be sure of the reasons for her decision, but the difficult atmosphere at Claybury during this period meant that female medical officers were very unlikely to be promoted. Remaining unemployed for the following few months, she continued to volunteer at the Canning Town Medical Mission, and when the superintendent there took extended sick leave in March, she was offered the role.

The superintendent position was a significant progression from her previous job, albeit in an institution with equally little prestige; the Medical Mission was a charitable out-patient dispensary for East London's working-class women and children. Nevertheless, the role provided an opportunity to gain valuable clinical experience in a wide range of medical problems, including nervous disorders. The medical mission gave Boyle the chance to observe insanity in its early stages, especially amongst poor patients where no proper institutional treatment could be offered until they worsened and were admitted to the county asylum (Boyle 1939). Doctors at the mission were often involved in care in the domestic environment, as the remit of the medical mission included 'free medical attention at the dispensary, nursing in the home, some care for the general welfare for the patients,' and in some cases, 'a hospital for those needing institutional treatment' (Heasman 1964, p. 231). For Boyle, seeing the patient not only in the hospital but in the home highlighted the connections between nervous disorder and the social problems caused by poverty, as well as the seemingly inevitable decline that resulted from delaying care (Westwood 2001). This reinforced what she had learnt at Claybury: that current state policy simply did not concern itself with mental disease until the individual had become certifiably insane and was thus actively contributing to the overcrowding of asylums and incurability of patients.

The position at Canning Town was temporary. Boyle left at the end of the year, moving to Brighton to establish her own general practice with her friend and colleague from Claybury, Dr Mabel Jones. In doing so, they became the first female GPs in Brighton and Hove (a significant professional success in itself) (Milliken 2010). In her practice, Boyle observed similar issues with working-class access to health care as she had in London (Westwood 2001). Alongside Jones, Boyle decided to use the knowledge she had gained at the medical mission and open a dispensary of her own. Boyle and Jones sought funding from well-to-do women in Brighton and the surrounding area; a community likely to approve of and support a charitable, woman-and-child focused venture such as theirs. By October 1899 they had secured the patronage of the Countess of Chichester and established a 'Council of Ladies' to oversee the running of an institution which would 'afford poor Women of Brighton and the Neighbourhood, the opportunity of Free Consultation with Doctors of their own Sex' (Annual Report of the Lewes Road Hospital and Lady Chichester Hospital and Dispensary [hereafter LCH Annual Report] 1900). The Lewes Road Dispensary for Women and Children (Under Medical Women) opened that year, with a staff of female physicians serving a population of 'laundry-workers and other poor women' (LCH Annual Report 1900). By the end of the first year of operation, over 1000 patients had signed onto the books.

In opening a medical institution for women, by women (from patients to medical staff to board members), Boyle was capitalising on the belief that there was special benefit in the same sex female patient-clinician relationship. Mary Ann Elston has charted the history of women's entry into the medical profession, demonstrating how the first generation of female doctors did not compete for 'equal rights' to men in the public sphere, 'but for access to it in order to better pursue their feminine interests and talents': the 'private domain of the family and personal philanthropy' (Elston 1986, p. 129). The 'notion of women as traditionally healers, and as guardians of both physical and moral family health, was developed to the conclusion that women should be doctors to those whose lives were based in the family' (Elston 1986, p. 134). Female physicians were *women* doctors specifically, 'bringing a distinctive vision to their work, one that drew on their distinctively female qualities' to effectively care for women and young children (Elston 1986, p. 135). Although the medical establishment and public supported this argument, it meant that the first women doctors were restricted to treating this demographic. In addition to the hostility and competition many women faced when applying for junior roles after medical school, there were few existing opportunities for women to treat only female patients. It was especially difficult for female doctors to get work in the large general hospitals, which would lead to lucrative consulting work in the future.

Consequently, many of the first generation of medical women set up their own women-only hospitals. Several of the women involved in the LSMW supported this mandate for women-only care, or at least saw its practical utility in furthering the medical woman's career. One of the founding council members, Elizabeth Garrett Anderson, had set up a dispensary for poor women and children in the 1860s, which later became the New Hospital for Women and Children. Likewise, one of the early graduates of the School, Dr Annie McCall, opened the Clapham Maternity Hospital in 1889, which was staffed by women and admitted female medical students only (A Clerical Correspondent 1889; Marks 1992; Elston 2001; Garrett Anderson 2016). Sophia Jex-Blake believed strongly in the moral value of female patients receiving treatment from a female doctor, arguing that 'the almost exclusive employment of physicians of their own sex' was an 'immense boon,' both 'physically and morally,' for 'suffering women' (Jex-Blake 1887). Boyle would have been exposed to these ideas, and the pioneering women who put them into practice, during her time at the LSMW. Given the difficulties that she had already faced attempting to work on a female ward within a male-dominated medical environment, we can see why Boyle would choose to follow in their footsteps and strike off in a separatist mode of practice. She was in good company.

Louise Westwood locates Boyle within a group of 'second-generation medical women' who used strategies of separation to 'enter new specialisms and achieve clinical autonomy' (Westwood 2006, pp. 92–93). She suggests that 'these goals were often realised by working in an all-female environment, and with children,' a career path which served to both carve out a specific role for women within medicine and 'ensure a measure of clinical freedom away from the competitive sphere of [mainstream practice] where women doctors faced unequal pay, patriarchy and poor career opportunities' (Westwood 2006, pp. 92–93). As Elston has argued, these separatist institutions were places where women could 'develop professional skills, and achieve positions of responsibility from which they were otherwise largely excluded, both by overt opposition and by the limited mandate' (Elston 1986, p. 220). Lewes Road was the beginning of Boyle's separatist approach; a path chosen because of its visible success for other women. The Lewes Road Dispensary did succeed, by 1904 offering almost 5,000 consultations to individual patients a year. Opening the Dispensary confirmed Boyle's belief in the 'value [women placed on] the opportunity of consulting Doctors of their own sex,' and shaped her approach to her professional future (LCH Annual Reports 1905). Boyle's next major career move was to utilise these separatist tactics to exploit a gap in the market in the care of the insane.

Boyle's experiences at Claybury and the Medical Mission were formative in developing her interest in insanity. In 1939 Boyle gave an address at an MPA meeting, recollecting on her career. In it she describes how her 'two and a half years as Assistant Medical Officer at Claybury Mental Hospital' and her superintendence at a 'little East End hospital' first made the need for early treatment clear to her, by highlighting how often patients were seen at both institutions (Boyle 1939, p. 863). She recalls how 'the East End supplied many of the patients I had been looking after at Claybury, and it was borne in upon me that here, still in their homes, were the patients already struggling under burdens which would subsequently overwhelm them, and which would bring them later, but often only much later, certified to Claybury' (Boyle 1939, p. 863). These experiences led her to the 'inescapable fact' that 'it was there and then [...] that they needed help and understanding treatment' (Boyle 1939, p. 863).

Unsurprisingly given the demographic of its patients, Lewes Road struggled with the same issues that Boyle found so prevalent at Canning Town. She saw how 'extremely difficult' it was to provide this help 'through ordinary philanthropic channels' (Boyle 1939, p. 860). General hospitals did not admit neurasthenic patients and successful treatment was not possible through outpatient care. These poor patients lacked the money to obtain the 'skilled treatment and discriminating supervision' necessary to prevent their later certification (Boyle 1939, p. 860).

At the turn of the century there were extremely limited facilities for the early treatment of nervous disorders, particularly for pauper and working-class patients. In her MPA address Boyle charts the development of early intervention in the pioneering work of a handful of mind doctors who set up outpatient facilities for nervous disorders around the country. The 'first great step [...] was taken by the late Dr Rayner' who 'acted upon his belief that patients in a mental hospital had often suffered for a long time before being admitted [...] and that by early treatment they might have recovered before reaching the stage at which they could be certified' (Boyle 1939, p. 860). Rayner therefore 'persuaded St. Thomas's Hospital to establish an out-patient department for them in 1889' (Boyle 1939, p. 860). He was followed by Dr Percy Smith, who worked at Bethlem; an institution which 'specialised in helping early cases' (Boyle 1939, p. 860). Smith later started the second out-patient clinic at Charing Cross Hospital. Provincial clinics were added by Dr Goodall at Cardiff Hospital and Dr Carswell at Glasgow Infirmary in the early twentieth century. The work of these men was strengthened by the campaigning of Sir Maurice Craig and Sir Frederick Mott, who had a direct influence on Boyle herself (Boyle 1839, pp. 860–863).

There were thus a vocal minority of campaigners for the early treatment of mental disease in the late nineteenth and early twentieth century and Boyle was not alone in wishing for reform, nor in campaigning for greater provision for the poor. However, existing facilities were few and far between, offering mainly outpatient care. Boyle saw an opportunity to expand Lewes Road and set up a much-needed inpatient facility. This facility, named the Lady Chichester Hospital after its patron, would provide treatment exclusively for women with non-certifiable mental disease. The new hospital met two previously disregarded needs: the early treatment of nervous disorders and psychiatric care for women by women.

The Lady Chichester Hospital for Women and Children: Reporting on a Separatist Approach

Emma Milliken (2010) has described the opening of the Lady Chichester in 1905. The hospital was run by the same committee of women which Boyle and Jones had gathered in 1899, the Vice-President of which was Elizabeth Garrett Anderson. Initially, the hospital had ten beds supervised by a Matron and two probationary staff, alongside Boyle and Jones themselves. It was funded by voluntary donations, fundraising by the committee, and by payment from patients (a small contribution to the costs of their care, dependent on what they could afford). Within a few years of its opening, the hospital had become popular enough that patients often had to wait for admission. Short wait times were crucial given the aims of early treatment and an expansion was planned. An anonymous donation in 1911 enabled the committee to proceed and in 1912 the hospital moved to new, larger premises with space for a total of 35 beds. That same year, Lewes Road was expanded and a general inpatients' hospital added to the dispensary and outpatients departments. By World War I, Boyle's facility had three distinct branches: an inpatients' hospital for nervous disorders, an inpatients' hospital for medical and surgical cases, and an outpatient department with a dispensary. All of these clinics were staffed and managed by women, providing, as Milliken has argued, a place where female doctors could 'improve their professional skills, increase their knowledge, and achieve positions of responsibility they were not able to achieve elsewhere' (Milliken 2010, p. 92).

The story of the Lady Chichester Hospital is told through the reports which were kept from the hospital's foundation until war broke out in 1914. These documents are institutional, yet they tell of Boyle's personal ambitions and the collective ethos under which she and her colleagues managed the hospital. Produced in November of each year, the reports include detailed accounts of the LCH, its aims, clinical practices, financial affairs, and council decisions. They were published, public facing documents, intended for consumption by audiences beyond those directly involved in the institution's management.[4] Such reports became common practice for charitable medical institutions during the nineteenth century.

[4] The annual reports were published in Brighton, by the Southern Publishing Company Ltd, London.

Annual reports communicated information about an institution's activities (over the preceding year) to stakeholders and the public, with the ostensible purpose of holding the board accountable for their actions.[5] However, these reports were also a useful tool for image management. William J. Jackson has described how for 'voluntary hospital managers [...] the primary objective was the maintenance of an image of scrupulous honesty, integrity and efficiency in the running of the affairs of the hospital' (Jackson 2012, p. 52) Avoidance of any scandal was key: 'public opprobrium would be matched by a drying up of charitable support' (Jackson 2012, p. 52). Hospital boards were therefore careful to present a positive image, 'manifested most powerfully in the form of the annual report' (Jackson 2012, p. 53). The reports were 'the primary interface between the hospitals and their communities' and were distributed amongst 'subscribers, churches, and other potential sources of finance, as well as to any other interested parties that requested a copy' (Jackson 2012, p. 54). As Patricia and John Stanton have argued, the annual reports were often treated as a publicity exercise by the board. They are texts which 'proactively construct a particular visibility and meaning, rather than revealing "what was there"' (Stanton and Stanton 2002, p. 478).

Boyle and the Lady Chichester committee appear to have been particularly aware of the potential value of these texts as a means to seek support (and donations) for their innovative hospital. The reports were a textual space over which Boyle had full control, enabling her to communicate her clinical vision to valuable audiences. Readers would have undoubtedly included wealthy members of the public, other physicians, and interested mind doctors. Boyle took advantage of the publicity provided by the annual reports to cultivate a positive professional image that both satisfied her desire for reform and ensured she did not alienate potential donors. Cleverly capitalising on the novel attribute of the hospital—that it was women-led—the annual reports displayed the Lady Chichester in the best possible light, in both their content and design.

The texts are beautiful objects, designed to be appealing to the reader. Tiny, palm-sized printed pamphlets, they have a decorative cover made of coloured card and embellished with a delicate ink border and curlicues. Inside, the typeface is neat and small, and the paper of good quality.

[5] For a useful overview of annual reports in the archive, the University of Hull Library has a helpful webpage: https://libguides.hull.ac.uk/common-record-types/annual-reports.

Although a professional document, the reports have a particular daintiness and intricacy; they are aesthetically pleasing where simple utility would usually suffice. This attractiveness of form conveys an image of genteel femininity which the reader would associate with the institution itself. The pamphlets thus hinted that the hospital and its female staff embodied a certain refinement and respectability idealised in middle-class women during this period. This was a considered, deliberate decision by Boyle and the LCH committee, a tactical gendering of clinical practice. The reports act as a brochure for the hospital and are a visual representation of the institution's ethos which Boyle and her colleagues outline in detail inside each pamphlet: the Lady Chichester was a professional, successful, welcoming and, importantly, feminine facility.

The annual reports outlined a manifesto for the hospital which argued that a female-centric approach to treatment was crucial. The first report, published just after the hospital opened in 1905, introduced the idea that 'unsuitable' environments had a significant part to play in the development of mental disease (LCH Annual Report 1905). These environmental factors were often specific to the domestic space. Such considerations were therefore very important in the treatment of women, who in most cases held all household and familial responsibilities; 'the constant pressure of modern life is felt by women of all classes alike' (LCH Annual Report 1910). As the 1911 report claimed, there were 'wives and mothers of families whose circumstances make it impossible for them to get rest or relief so long as they remain in their own homes' (LCH Annual Report 1911). The only chance of recovery they had was to be taken away from 'the daily strain' (LCH Annual Report 1911). The reports argued that the LCH was the best place to help these women get well.

Patients would have access to top female medical staff; a 'House Surgeon, a specially trained and experienced Matron, and two Probationers,' who 'devote themselves constantly' to the care of their charges (LCH Annual Report 1906). There were varied treatments, from 'complete bed rest' to 'abundant outdoor exercise,' 'electric and hydropathic' facilities and 'massage,' administered as each patient required (LCH Annual Report 1906). Most crucial to the LCH's methodology, however, was the special homely atmosphere patients would experience. No effort was 'spared to make the daily life at the Hospital bright and interesting,' and as 'home-like as possible' (LCH Annual Report 1906). A 'good tone and happy relations' was maintained at all times amongst residents (LCH Annual Report 1909). Patients were encouraged to participate in the regular routine of the hospital as much as they were able, 'assisting[ing] in housework' and providing entertainment for the more poorly patients (LCH Annual Report 1909). In turn, they were encouraged to take an active part in the warm, welcoming community with 'music,' 'suitable home-occupations' and 'games' always available to them (LCH Annual Report 1905).

This philosophy had strong echoes of moral treatment practices, with its emphasis on the institution as family and the psychological benefits of a restful, healthy lifestyle. Boyle and the Lady Chichester committee had dispensed with the paternalism of these ideas, however, and created a feminised version of moral management. The LCH replicated the privacy, trust, and domestic environment of the Victorian treatment regime but officered entirely by female staff, adapted them to support a separatist ideal built on the innate benefits of care by women. The reports argued that the cure for incipient nervous disease was to extract the sufferer from the environment which was causing them harm and allow them to recover in a specially controlled replication of the perfect home. Female doctors were doubly suited to provide patients with the treatment they so badly needed; as women, the physicians of the Lady Chichester were qualified to offer both medical assistance *and* domestic care.

Both the design and content of the annual reports sell a vision of the female alienist, built on contemporary expectations about the female gender and women's special skills and capacities. This was a strategy which promoted an acceptable face of the institution and supported its separatist approach, without alienating either the public or the medical mainstream. These texts demonstrate how Boyle and her colleagues manipulated late-nineteenth century ideologies of femininity, visually and discursively, to produce a narrative which minimised the challenge to the status quo that their unusual clinical practices represented. Boyle was keenly aware of the power of textual form when deployed as an advertising tool, using feminised language and imagery to suggest that there was a niche in the psychiatric marketplace that only women were able to fill. Crucially, she intentionally made use of these texts to deliver a rhetoric which would allow her to further her career.

Unlike in other medical specialties, female-led practice was unusual in the treatment of insanity and nervous disorders; Boyle's focus on women was unique, not just in early treatment, but in psychiatry. As Charlotte Mackenzie (1983) has demonstrated, whilst women sometimes led the care of the insane prior to its professionalisation (for example, as proprietors of private madhouses), by the late nineteenth century they were marginalised within the discipline. In county asylums like Claybury, 'women remained in the lower ranks of the profession' (Mackenzie 1983, p. 118). When employed, they were only allowed to supervise the female wards and 'promotion to more senior positions was barred by their lack of experience on male wards' (Mackenzie 1983, p. 118). Senior women in public asylums (matrons and housekeepers) 'were subject to the authority of medical superintendents' who were always male (Mackenzie 1983, p. 117). The Lady Chichester Hospital was different as it enabled Boyle to operate outside of these restrictions.

It is perhaps because of the revolutionary nature of the LCH that the reports were at pains to explain how the hospital was of benefit not only for its patients but for society. The texts emphasised that inexpensive, early inpatient treatment for the poor was necessary, as they had no alternative. These patients were unable to 'afford an expensive rest-cure,' and any treatment at home was 'apt to be rendered ineffective by wrong conditions' (LCH Annual Report 1906). Whether 'depressing surroundings,' the toil of hard work, or 'want of proper nourishment and comfort,' poverty had a direct impact on the progress of nervous disorders (LCH Annual Report 1906). It was likely that the individual would worsen under these conditions to the point where they would 'fall out of the ranks of workers, too often becoming a burden on the rates' as pauper asylum patients (LCH Annual Report 1910). This was especially tragic for women as 'the comfort and happiness of entire families' depended on them (LCH Annual Report 1910). 'Complete breakdown' of the mother might even mean 'permanent handicap of the children whom she has to bring up and control' (LCH Annual Report 1911). Institutions like the Lady Chichester were vital for the sake of future generations: it was 'most important for the country that these women should receive whatever they require to prevent their ultimate collapse' (LCH Annual Report 1911).

The language of these reports draws on gendered ideas of women's place in the home, national pride, and the dangers and pressures of modern life to promote an institutional ideal of rest and recuperation. Boyle's argument that patients required a clinically simulated domestic environment to get well justified her in taking them out of their homes and away from the duties of family and work which she believed were actively causing them harm. Enclosing the patient in the institution, she temporarily absolved women of these responsibilities so that they could return to society as useful members of the household. As the 1905 report proudly stated, 'the large number of patients treated during the past year (1,642 patients, 4,984 consultations) affords continued proof of the fact that poor women greatly value the opportunity of consulting Doctors of their own sex' (LCH Annual Report 1905).

These were powerful and persuasive ideas. The reports utilised established beliefs about the special role of women doctors to justify the need for a female-run psychiatric hospital. The old tropes of women's caring and delicate nature, previously held as reasons why they might be unsuited to the management of lunatics, were presented as explanations for exactly why they in fact should take on this responsibility. In arguing for the usefulness of women doctors based on these gendered characteristics, Boyle made it very difficult for potential critics to contest her views; to do so, they would have to contradict the very gendered ideas they espoused. The specialist treatment of women who carry the moral responsibility of home and society on their shoulders gave the LCH a mandate to operate. A discursive textual space associated in the medical and public mind with charitable, reputable institutions (where supportive patient data and financial figures could also be provided) was the ideal form in which Boyle might put forward these arguments.

For Boyle, the key benefit of the LCH was that it enabled her to run her own hospital, which gave her the freedom to design her own clinical methodology. Her decision to treat incipient nervous disorders stemmed from a desire to effect change in clinical methods that she felt hamstrung contemporary state provision for the insane. In choosing to set up her own institution for women and children, she was capitalising on her identity as a woman to create a space outside of the patriarchal asylum system, in which she could put her theories into practice. Boyle's approach to treatment was quite unlike the practices seen in asylums in Britain at the time, not only because of her intention to effect cure at an early stage of mental disease, but also because she combined a wide range of environmental, social, psychological and biological approaches to mental illness.

By the turn of the century, most British mind doctors had narrowed their clinical focus to psychopathology (Clark 1981; Berrios and Freeman 1991; Shorter 1998; Roelcke et al. 2010). Jennifer Wallis has shown how late nineteenth-century alienists were interested in 'research that aimed to uncover the bodily root of mental disease,' undertaking 'microscopic investigations of brain tissue and nerve cells, or attempts to link physical and mental anomalies with discrete lesions of the brain substance' (Wallis

2017, pp. 1–2). The Lady Chichester Hospital did not have the means to set up a pathological laboratory like that at Claybury and in any case Boyle resisted the localisation of the psychopathological model and drew on multifarious theories of the mind. Emma Milliken describes Boyle's clinical practice as a 'holistic psycho-biological' (Milliken 2010, p. 221) methodology which recognised the 'close interdependence between the social environment in which people lived, and the development of mental illness' (Milliken 2010, p. 216); an approach no doubt influenced by her work at Canning Town and Lewes Road. Milliken suggests that Boyle instead used 'observation and common sense' (Milliken 2010, p. 224) to create 'an individual psychology, a merger of all the theories and treatments she found convincing, with a complete disregard for any she did not' (Milliken 2010, p. 238).

Particularly significant for the treatment of women with mental disorders, this holistic approach meant that the Lady Chichester Hospital did not place any special emphasis on the reproductive function of the female body. As the LCH annual reports show, the hospital focused on the 'provision of skilled treatment, care, rest, and good feeding,' alongside the clinical benefits of 'open-air life' and 'suitable home-occupations' (LCH Annual Report 1905). These practices were intended to combat the 'worry, over-work, and insufficient food' which Boyle saw as the true aggravating factors of nervous disease (LCH Annual Report 1905). Like the women correspondents who replied to Maudsley in the periodical press three decades previously, Boyle did not explicitly dismiss gynaecological treatment or argue against the validity of the connection made between female reproductive organs and the mind. Instead, she stressed the impact of women's social, domestic, and working lives on their minds, downplaying the importance of the reproductive connection in the maintenance of female mental health by simply declining to address the issue. Indeed, in one of the cases given in the annual reports, a lady 'broken down after the climacteric' is treated merely by 'rest, feeding up, medicines, encouragement and reassurance' (LCH Annual Report 1913).

This emphasis on the social causes of nervous disease is reflected in the admissions registers kept from the hospital's opening in 1905. These registers were intended to chart the admission and discharge of patients arriving at the hospital and to record important information about them pertinent to their care. Patients were recorded in order of admission, their details entered in a table which included categories such as name, address, occupation, age, who recommended them for admission, the person responsible for the patient, dates of admission and discharge, weight on admission and discharge, and which disorder they suffered from. Admissions registers were just one of the many clinical records used in asylums to classify and manage large patient populations (Craig 1991; Risse and Warner 1992; Bynum 1994; Lorkowski and Pokorski 2022). As discussed in Chapter 4, the registers were often referred to in patients' case notes and provided the foundation for decisions made about where patients were housed in the institution and what type of treatment was embarked upon. As such, they were texts which had a structural function within the asylum, organising patients both conceptually (for example, as manic or demented) and physically.

At the Lady Chichester the staff appear to have been quite lax at keeping patient data. For much of the period until 1914, the records entered for each patient are incomplete, with many of the fields left blank. The disorder the patient was suffering from, for example, often went unrecorded, as did the staff member responsible for them after admission. There was thus a resistance of, or at least apathy to, the clinical classifications the registers encourage. Interestingly, the field for occupation *was* completed for every patient: the register carefully records the job each woman did, from housewife to domestic servant, to teacher or dressmaker (LCH Register of Patients 1904–1910 and 1910–1914).

The Lady Chichester Hospital endeavoured to provide care for the poorer women in society and the registers would have been a method of monitoring which class of people were admitted to the hospital. However, the focus on occupation (as opposed to income, relevant for the charging of the hospital's discretionary fees) indicates that this data had additional significance for Boyle and her staff. The diligence with which patient occupation was input into the register suggests that it was felt to be germane to their illness, a way for the staff to track how social environment precipitated the onset of nervous disorders. We know from the LCH annual reports that Boyle believed strongly in the impact of social factors in mental disease, in particular the effect which the difficult living conditions of working-class women had on their health. These records demonstrate that a causal link was being made between living conditions and admission, and imply that there was a clinical focus on social aetiology. In contrast, gynaecological theories of women's madness relied on a physiological and pathological approach to mental illness and its treatment. The admissions registers are further evidence that the reproductive interpretation of female insanity was of little use to Boyle in her psycho-social treatment regime.

The founding of the Lady Chichester Hospital facilitated Boyle's career progression by enabling her to reach a position of greater professional authority (as founder and chief honourable medical officer) than she had previously achieved. This professional authority in turn allowed her to fulfil a further aim: independence and innovation in her clinical practice. She could not achieve these aims from inside the asylum system because of the lack of power afforded to physicians of her gender. Boyle's separationist tactics were thus extremely useful in providing her with the professional opportunities she desired. However, the Lady Chichester annual reports demonstrate that Boyle was cautious not to alienate herself from others in the field. Remaining a part of the professional community of practicing mind doctors was as important to Boyle as her clinical independence.

Early Treatment in the *Journal of Mental Science*: Boyle's Inclusionist Approach

Although Louise Westwood suggests that Boyle was a 'separatist pioneer,' Boyle courted and achieved professional integration in several key areas of her working life, most significantly in her membership of the MPA (Westwood 2006, p. 93). The MPA was founded as the Association of Medical Officers of Asylums and Hospitals for the Insane in 1841, transforming to the rather less wordy Medico-Psychological Association in 1865. It was an organisation created to represent those qualified to work in the care of the insane and to further research into mental illness, and by the 1890s had nearly 600 members. It remained the only medical society devoted to psychiatry well into the twentieth century and membership was key for those wishing to work within the field (Turner 1991; Renvoize 1991). Formed at a time when the discipline was carving a space for itself in the medical community, the MPA was an attempt to professionalise and define the boundaries of psychiatry, within which its members could claim to operate. This reflected wider changes in medical practice, which became increasingly specialised during this period (Weisz 2003). In effect, the MPA functioned like many other medical and scientific societies of the Victorian era, running meetings and debates for its members to discuss new theories, lobbying for legislative or other forms of change in the field, and publishing the *Journal of Mental Science*. The *JMS* featured original articles on insanity (which were mostly papers from MPA meetings), clinical cases, reviews, asylum reports, coverage of recently published research, and notes on meetings and newsworthy items.

Boyle joined the MPA in 1898 when she moved to Brighton to set up her general practice. Membership of the Association had been open to women for only four years, and she was one of only a handful to have membership.[6] The MPA was in fact one of the first medical societies to admit female members. Until the late nineteenth century, women working in medicine were largely excluded from participating in the professionalisation and development of their chosen field, as the meetings and journals run by these societies both directed and consolidated disciplinary practice. For Boyle, joining the MPA would therefore have been a significant act. It was a declaration that she was a professional in the mind sciences and a symbol of belonging important to her own identity formation as a female doctor. Yet it was also, in practical terms, a method of gaining access to the workings of the field. Although Boyle was willing to operate outside of traditional asylum structures through necessity, it seems she still wanted her ideas to be heard by the medical establishment. Boyle was an active participant in the Association. She remained a member of the MPA for the duration of her career, making such a name for herself in the discipline that she became the first female president in 1939.

That Boyle was so involved in the society's proceedings indicates that belonging to this professional body aligned with her own career aspirations and was a measure of achievement for her. As one of very few practicing women mind doctors, belonging to the MPA must have been validating and affirming: her right to practise was officially recognised through her membership to the organisation. Boyle's career path suggests that she was ambitious, in some respects in an orthodox fashion. In later life, she took on many advisory and honorary positions of prestige in medical institutions, including becoming a member of the council of psychiatry at the Royal Society of Medicine in 1928, as well as an honorary consultant in nervous disease at the Royal Sussex Hospital in 1930 (the first woman to hold an honorary position at that hospital). She also helped to found further professional bodies, such as the National Council of Mental Hygiene (later MIND) (Milliken 2006). Boyle's

[6] Emma Milliken (2010) identifies 17 women who were employed in psychiatry before 1900. Of these, 13 were members of the MPA.

membership of the MPA helped her progress to these roles, as it was a valuable ally in both allowing her to build a useful network of colleagues and in normalising her separatist actions, which may have otherwise hindered mainstream medicine's acceptance of her methods.

She also made several contributions to the *Journal of Mental Science*. Boyle's first article was a 'Case of Juvenile Paralysis', published in 1899 (Boyle 1899). She went on to publish a further four papers in the journal. Three of these, published between the founding of the LCH and World War I, deal with the hospital's treatment practices and ethos: the rather similarly titled 'Some Points in the Early Treatment of Mental and Nervous Cases (with Special Reference to the Poor)' (Boyle 1905), 'Account of an Attempt at the Early Treatment of Mental and Nervous Cases (with Special Reference to the Poor)' (Boyle 1909), and 'Some Observations on Early Nervous and Mental Cases, with Suggestions as to Possible Improvement in our Methods of Dealing with Them' (Boyle 1914). These texts promote Boyle's theories of early treatment and demonstrate the value of the LCH to the Association. They are therefore evidence of an inclusionist tactic which, whilst complementary, remained distinct from Boyle's approach in the reports.

These publications were an important method which Boyle used to cultivate an intellectual relationship with her peers. By the end of the nineteenth century, medical journals were vital to the communication of clinical and scientific findings, and the formation of scientific communities (Shuttleworth and Charnely 2016; Dawson et al. 2020). Alex Csiszar has shown how 'the modern scientific journal is largely an invention of the nineteenth century,' during which period 'the scientific paper' became 'the chief avenue by which to make the results of [...] research into public knowledge claims' (Csiszar 2018, p. 4). The scientific journal became 'widely accepted' as a 'special class of publications that could be demarcated from other forms of periodical literature' (Csiszar 2018, p. 5). They became 'purveyors of scientific news but also archives of discovery,' legitimising practitioner's research findings and generating scientific reputation (Csiszar 2018, p. 8). As Csiszar has argued, 'scientific authority was reconfigured around periodical authorship and reading' (Csiszar 2018, p. 18). If Boyle wished to share her ideas with her colleagues (and importantly, do so on an equal footing), such a periodical was a very useful avenue of communication.

Boyle's publications for the *JMS* are written records of papers which she gave to delegates at quarterly and annual MPA meetings. In giving these papers, Boyle was actively participating in the culture of the MPA. She was also producing a written record of her theories which, alongside her name, was widely shared. Such exposure was a good measure of professional prestige and established a reputation which Boyle could (and did) utilise in the future. The peculiarity of Boyle's works for the *JMS* is that as dual texts, existing as both speech and written essay, they had a particularly varied reach. In presenting her papers to the MPA, Boyle was able to engage with her audience twice over: in the moment, as a doctor standing before her peers, and again (and again) as her published text was circulated amongst readers of the journal. Aware that her voice would be recorded on the page, Boyle must have known that her ideas would reach both the listeners in front of her and a wider community beyond. She was therefore speaking, not just to the handful of mind doctors present at the meeting, but to the hidden audience of the *JMS*. This audience included more of the MPA's 600 members, medical professionals outside of the specialism, and even interested members of the public.[7] If Boyle could convince them that her novel techniques were scientifically sound, she could boost the reputation of the LCH amongst her peers and gain further support to evolve her work.

Michael Shepherd (1992) has demonstrated how the *JMS* was the primary journal for the British psychiatric establishment during the nineteenth and early twentieth centuries. In fact, the *JMS*'s only competitors were *The Journal of Psychological Medicine and Mental Pathology* (1848–1883), which covered the psychology and philosophy of mind, and *Brain* (1878-Present), which increasingly focused on neurology and neurophysiology. The placement of Boyle's papers within the *JMS* thus did much to legitimise her more progressive views. The act of publication itself, in the major journal of psychiatry, was a move which confirmed her inclusion in the mainstream of the profession at the same time as it engineered it.

Specialist periodicals like the *JMS* were key to the formation of professional identity. As Michael Brown (2011) has shown, over the nineteenth century medical practitioners' sense of identity became increasingly based on claims to expertise. An overcrowded medical marketplace called for

[7] The *JMS* is mentioned and consulted in several periodicals from the popular press. For example, 'Feigned Insanity' in *Chambers's Journal* (1883) and 'Special Correspondence' in *British Architect* (1886) both cite the *JMS* as a source for information on insanity. Adverts for the *JMS* also appeared in non-specialist periodicals, such as the *Academy* and *Athenaeum*.

a new way to differentiate practitioners: through specialisation and disciplinarity (Weisz 2003). Periodicals were one of the primary ways in which these disciplinary identities were formed and enacted. As Alison Moulds has argued, 'practitioners used their writing to participate in acts of self-definition and to fashion ideas about their colleagues and rivals, as well as the wider profession' (Moulds 2021, p 3). Journals targeted at specific audiences helped to carve out the boundaries of different professional groups, and specialist periodicals 'dominated the field from the 1870s onwards' (Moulds 2021, p. 4). Professional memberships, and authorship in the journals controlled by these medical societies, were 'constructed as an important part of one's medical identity' (Moulds 2021, p. 176).

The *JMS* was first published in 1853 and originally edited by John Charles Bucknill (of textbook fame). It was published by John (later J&A) Churchill, which produced much of the psychiatric literature available on the market during the Victorian period (Chapter 2). Each number offered up-to-date coverage of the news and views of the elite of the discipline. Suzy Anger (2009) describes how, aside from the publication of MPA speeches and a smattering of essays from prominent scientists working on the brain (such as neurologist John Hughlings Jackson), much of the content of the *JMS* appears to have been written anonymously by its editors or their close professional associates. Henry Maudsley, Thomas Smith Clouston, George Henry Savage, and Daniel Hack Tuke were all at the helm of the *JMS* at various points during the nineteenth century. All regularly contributed material to the periodical. The journal was therefore the product of an intellectual elite of mind doctors strongly associated with the MPA, who worked at a small collection of asylums and published treatises and textbooks under Churchill, and who had a significant interest in promoting a particular image of their profession.

Boyle's writing for the *JMS* allowed her to fashion herself as part of this exclusive group. Excluded from the state asylum system, Boyle's membership of the MPA and authorship in the *JMS* were key to her ability to make connections with the psychiatric establishment. In fact, writing for the journal was the primary way in which she, as an outsider and a woman, could communicate with and influence her male colleagues. Despite this, Moulds has shown how the medical press was a 'predominantly masculine textual space, in which the editors, contributors, correspondents, and readers were typically male' (Moulds 2021, p. 182). Women's voices were 'mediated and often undermined' (Moulds 2021, p. 182). Although the

MPA admitted female members, Boyle was on the fringes of this little club and needed to be tactical to gain their acceptance.

Anger recounts how the *JMS* was initially intended to focus on 'practical issues such as mental physiology, mental disease and other matters important to "medical men who were engaged in the treatment of the insane"' (Anger 2009, p. 325). However, it was also hoped that the periodical would convey to the wider medical public that 'physicians dealing with mental illness require specialised medical training' (Anger 2009, p. 325). Professionalisation of the mind sciences was a key topic championed within its pages. Boyle appears to have gleaned this from her experiences of the MPA and employment in the field, as her arguments for the early treatment of nervous disorders are couched in these ideas. Her periodical publications demonstrate how she made strategic use of her textual platform by playing to the discipline's needs and concerns, appealing to the interests of asylum clinicians as well as arguing for her beliefs. Boyle's first two papers on the Lady Chichester present the hospital as an example of advancing professionalisation. In these articles she leaves behind the focus on gender and female-led care which we find in the LCH reports, to employ a rhetoric which emphasises the social and moral duty of psychiatry to better assist those suffering with mental illness. Crucially, Boyle argues that the provision of inpatient care should be extended through 'the establishment throughout the country of institutions for the treatment of nervous cases and of early uncertifiable insanity' (Boyle 1905, p. 676).

In 'Some Points' (1905) and 'Account of an Attempt' (1909), Boyle aligns her vision of extended care for the mentally ill with the values of expertise, social progress, and national service. In her 1905 paper, written just as the LCH was founded, Boyle suggests that the absence of facilities for early treatment has resulted in patients being 'forced into insanity or a nervous condition from which there might be no recovery possible,' either to 'live an incubus upon the rates' or 'probably to die' (Boyle 1905, p. 677). This state of affairs, she argues, 'seems hardly like a civilised nation' (Boyle 1905, p. 677). The 'same England' that does so much in the 'prevention of cruelty to children and to animals' allows so many of its 'good workers to be driven into insanity for want of timely and suitable aid' (Boyle 1905, p. 678). Boyle here touches on the major problems faced in the management of the insane at the turn of the twentieth century: the incurability of patients leading to both the costly overburdening of the asylum system and the loss of productive members of society to a disease which left them debilitated for many years. Boyle urges the reader, 'for the sake of humanity and the economy' to support the establishment of hospitals for the treatment of these unfortunate patients (Boyle 1905, p. 681). She cleverly combines a call to the alienist to prevent suffering (appealing to the doctor's wish to cure) with a solution to a practical issue which was dogging the profession and making it increasingly unpopular in wider society: the bloated asylum population. Early treatment was more likely to lead to patient recovery and avoidance of the asylum altogether.

In her 1909 paper, Boyle presses home the continued necessity of preventing 'mental patients being manufactured from the rough' by lack of state provision of care (Boyle 1909, p. 684). Nervous disease is a question of national health. Boyle argues that it is 'too common [...] to be safe' left untreated and is responsible for 'much crime and unemployment' (Boyle 1909, p. 685). 'There seems to be no question of more imminent social and national importance, none more worthy of discussion' than how to remedy nervous strain when the spectre of 'national degeneration' loomed large (Boyle 1909, p. 684). In this paper, written well into the first decade of the twentieth century, Boyle addresses concerns over the health of the British population, which had been festering since the time of Maudsley's 'Sex in Mind and in Education.' By the turn of the century, the idea that civilisation was making people unwell (or conversely, that some people were unfit for civilised society) had taken root. The eugenics movement had gained traction in intellectual and medical circles, and nervous weakness was feared to be transmitted down through generations (Saunders 1988; Pick 1989; Richardson 2003).

Philippa Levine and Alison Bashford have described how eugenics 'rapidly became a shared language and ambition' across locations, cultures, and movements (Levine and Bashford 2012, p. 2), emerging as a 'distinct theory in the 1880s' and thriving in the years around the First World War (Levine and Bashford 2012, p. 9). The 'aim of most eugenics movements was to affect reproductive practice through the application of theories of heredity', to influence the evolution of human populations through selective breeding (Levine and Bashford 2012, p. 1). Early twentieth-century eugenicists operated in an environment of 'widespread nationalisation [...] and new ways of thinking about populations as a citizenry, as a labour force, and as the generator of future fitness' (Levine and Bashford 2012, p. 2). Drawing on the work of Francis Galton, eugenicists envisioned interventionist techniques such as reproductive control and segregation, aiming to engineer healthier future generations. In psychiatry, as Mathew Thomson has shown, fears centred on the feebleminded and chronically insane: individuals possessed of a 'mental (and thus social) inadequacy' detrimental to the fostering of 'national efficiency in an era of escalating international competition' (Thomson 2012, p. 4). In Britain, the Mental Deficiency Act of 1913 allowed for a 'new system of institutions for the "feebleminded,"' due to the concern that disability 'would spread [through inheritance] unless this population was confined' (Thomson 2012, p. 3).

In her 1909 article Boyle placed early treatment in its national context. The mental health of society was now just as important as that of the individual patient and the treatment of nervous disorders was a necessary component of social health. However, Boyle did not write extensively on eugenics and there is no evidence that she either subscribed to the movement's views or implemented their policies. Her discussion of these ideas may have been an attempt to play to her readers, recognising and utilising contemporary discussions in the *JMS* to emphasise how crucial early treatment was. In fact, in 1913 she took steps to prevent the permanent institutionalisation of the mentally disabled under the new Act by setting up the Brighton Guardianship Society, a charity which aimed to provide care in the community for the feebleminded. Boyle believed that the key issue, in all but congenital cases, was timely intervention by an appropriate professional (Boyle 1939).

Boyle suggests that the mind doctor should have complete superiority in the management of the insane. She argues that the alienist is the only individual qualified to determine the right course of action, both individually in patient care, and nationally in policy. Early nervous disorder is a 'truth which terribly needs to be driven and hammered into the understanding of the lay public, and even more into that of the general practitioner, who is too apt to associate mental trouble with the striking picture of an acute maniac' (Boyle 1905, p. 676). Here Boyle reaffirms the disciplinary boundaries of psychiatry as a necessary specialism which meets a diagnostic and therapeutic need unable to be fulfilled by general practice. Alienists could identify those 'rescuable cases' who might be saved by the intervention of their professional expertise (Boyle 1905, p. 677). Significantly, she argues for this intervention to occur earlier than the state system of care for the insane allowed: before the patient was certified insane and admitted to the asylum. Treatment by experts 'was only attainable after they had [...] become sufficiently disordered in their conduct to need physical control' (Boyle 1909, p. 684). Yet 'any alienist knows the signs, so slight to those who are not interested [...] which herald a breakdown, and herald it too often uselessly for months and sometimes for years' (Boyle 1909, p. 684). Certification, she contended, was 'only an incident in the course of the insane illness, and not necessarily, nor even often, at the beginning of it' (Boyle 1905, p. 676). Once the patient had reached the asylum and its team of mind doctors, it was often too late for a cure.

Boyle frames the introduction of early treatment as an extension of the professional remit of psychiatry; a clear example of the disciplinary development that the MPA and its members supported. After the 1845 Lunacy Act, for a patient to be admitted to an asylum they had to be certified insane by two medical professionals. Boyle agrees that the law was 'a very valuable one,' seeing that physical control, when given, is not abused (Boyle 1905, p. 676). However, the Act also set the limits of the psychiatric profession. Certification represented the moment at which medical care for the insane legally began. In 1890, a further Act was passed which also made certification a requirement for patients at private madhouses, further regulating alienist involvement in early cases and discouraging financially able patients from seeking help from these institutions due to the stigma of certification (Takabayashi 2017). This represented a significant infringement on the professional freedoms of the mind-doctoring community as it narrowed both their area of practice and a lucrative income stream that many physicians relied upon alongside their posts at public asylums. Boyle challenges the process of certification by arguing for private and charitable, institutional early intervention. This would bypass these regulations and allow the mind doctor access to the patient at a stage of the disease where they might have the power to help (conveniently expanding the reach of the discipline at the same time).

In this context, Boyle's own separatist approach was not only valid but required; a model of care outside of the asylum that should be adopted wholesale across England. When Boyle draws attention to the Lady Chichester, it is to support these theories of early treatment and provide an example for others in the profession to follow. She describes the features and policies of her institution so that they may be emulated by other doctors wishing to set up their own hospitals. In 'Some Points' she describes the policy that 'patients are not kept in bed unless needful for their health,' and that 'the medical supervision is done by people who have had some experience of both insanity and neurology' (Boyle 1905, p. 679). 'Account of an Attempt…' covers staffing arrangements, costs, and cure rates, as well as outlining a treatment plan which attempts to teach 'that mental hygiene' which will safeguard patients from future collapse (Boyle 1909, pp. 686–687). Although any discussion of gender is otherwise absent, Boyle does suggest that there 'should be provision for the treatment of women by women' (Boyle 1905, p. 681). Her tone is less polemical than in the Chichester reports as she justifies this position in a rather tongue-in-cheek fashion: 'I may be forgiven for thinking that this is often a help to the patients. It is easier for a woman to understand a woman and the things that she does not say than it is for a man to do so; and though no doubt there are cases where it will be as well not to understand too much, a certain amount of density is easily assumed' (Boyle 1905, p. 681). Boyle is of course recognising her audience with these words.

In 1914, in the months leading up to the First World War, Boyle gave what would be her last paper for the MPA for many years. Published in the *JMS* in July, 'Some Observations' continues to push for further professionalisation and expansion of treatment for early nervous and mental cases. Boyle encourages the development of facilities for these patients, as well as improved education on nervous disorders for medical students. Even after the study of mental disease became a compulsory part of the medical curriculum in 1893, nervous cases were not amongst the patients on the psychiatric wards in general teaching hospitals. Boyle argues that such cases would never be 'efficiently understood' until this were to change: 'the cases which it seems to me all-important for students to see and study, are not the delirium tremens, the acute mania, the certifiable cases, but rather the early uncertifiable ones, the obsessional, the early melancholic, the hysterical' (Boyle 1914, p. 387). Not only were separate institutions required for the treatment of these patients, but some degree of integration of the specialism into mainstream medicine. Perhaps rather to the contrary, Boyle also sought to defend the alienist's position against an onslaught of inappropriately trained rival practitioners. She lists a total of fourteen different groups attempting the treatment of nervous disorders, from GPs to Christian scientists and occultists, before remarking indignantly: 'In fact, who generally does not see [an early mental case] at all, until and unless it has become certifiable? The Alienist' (Boyle 1914, p. 383).

She also addresses the tension between neurology and psychiatry that resutled from disputes over the comparative definitions of mental and nervous disease, and the physiological origins of insanity. Towards the end of the nineteenth century the study of the somatic causes of mental disease became increasingly popular, particularly in German psychiatry (Shorter 1998; Engstrom 2003). This encouraged an appreciation of the role of the nerves in insanity. As Akinobu Takabayashi has shown, 'neurologists played a significant role in the post-1890 psychiatric market' (Takabayashi 2017, p. 257). Interested 'primarily in physiological aspects of the nerve rather than pathological ones,' they did also see 'mild mental cases' in their private clinics (Takabayashi 2017, p. 257). This resulted in competition between the two fields and tension arose between physicians practising neurology and those working with the insane.

Arguing that 'early nervous and mental cases are inseparable in the abstract, and still more inseparable in practice,' Boyle suggests that treatment will only truly be efficacious when the two fields are combined (Boyle 1914, p. 381). Any 'arbitrary artificial separation is unscientific, and productive of mistakes and misunderstandings fatal to their [...] treatment, and [...] correct scientific appraisement and investigation' (Boyle 1914, p. 381). A proper understanding of the two specialisms would lead the doctor to accurately decide the case, particularly as 'all the physical signs we used to rely on for the diagnosis of organic nervous disease have now been described as existing in functional cases' (Boyle 1915, p. 387). Boyle argues simply, 'if all neurologists were alienists too' then there would be far better hope of finding cures for more types of mental disease (Boyle 1914, p. 385). Boyle was interested in keeping up with the latest scientific thought in her field and had toured the German *kliniks* when preparing to open the LCH. Visiting Ziehen, Kraepelin, and Cramer's institutions she was impressed by their 'grand possibilities for research, treatment and teaching'; like Claybury they combined laboratory work with patient care (Boyle 1905, p. 678). Drawing on these experiences abroad and perhaps influenced by her maverick, holistic attitude to treatment, Boyle could see the value in combining disciplines. She was able to conceive of a transformative vision for early treatment, as always situating her practice within the changing concerns of the profession to ensure a receptive audience in the MPA.

Writing these long form speeches-cum-essays, Boyle had the opportunity to engage in a discursive style that emphasised her expertise and professionalism. These articles reveal Boyle's considerable skills in rhetoric, as she marries her ambitions and clinical interests with the profession's needs. The rhetoric of her MPA papers was certainly playing to her audience but Boyle was not insincere. Boyle's publications for the *JMS* demonstrate not that she altered her attitudes based on her audience but that she was able to alter the justification for them to achieve support in different corners. Her papers for the *JMS* required her to speak to the concerns of a specialist professional audience, narrower than that of the annual reports of her hospital. She therefore needed to place her institution in a context that reflected the issues that troubled the alienist community. These papers are evidence of Boyle's awareness of the shifting pressures of her role within the discipline and highlight her skill in positioning herself for success as a woman in the medical marketplace.

Boyle tactfully harnessed the power of textual communication in her journey of self-promotion and adapted her language and content to suit her readership. Writing directly to members of her discipline, she not only showed sensitivity to their professional concerns but took full advantage of the opportunity to display her clinical knowledge to receptive specialists in the field. Publishing a medical paper was itself a marker of expertise which furthered her career in the mind sciences. Boyle contributed to the *JMS* at a period in which women were able to participate in published medical discourse for the first time, as newly qualified female doctors gradually gained membership to the medical societies which ran and published these specialist journals. Recognising the importance of writing to the professional reputation of male alienists, Boyle was something of a pioneer in her decision to utilise publication in support of her integration as a woman doctor.

Conclusion

Unusually for medical societies at the time, the MPA began publishing the debates from its meetings alongside members' papers from 1907 onwards. The latter two of Boyle's articles have these discussions attached. Filtered through the minute keeper's hands as well as editorial decisions on which remarks to keep for posterity, the responses are nevertheless as close to a verbatim account of what members thought about Boyle's theories on early treatment as is available to us. Interestingly, they demonstrate how far such theories had come to be valued since Boyle's struggles at Claybury and Canning Town. Members praised 'Dr Boyle's pioneer work' and hoped that her institution would be 'imitated all over the country, for need of it was very great indeed' (Boyle 1909, p. 691). They agreed that 'the Association ought to make a special acknowledgement to Dr Helen Boyle for the magnificent work she had done in the face of what must be recognised as enormous difficulties' (Boyle 1909, p. 691). Her 'rational methods of treatment' were very much supported (Boyle 1909, p. 691).

Boyle was a key pioneer in the campaign for early treatment of nervous disorders in Britain, a fact acknowledged here by her colleagues. The interest shown by members indicates that they were convinced by her arguments for further institutional development. No objection was made based on her sex, either to the aptitude Boyle had for her work or the worthiness of her theories. In so far as Boyle's inclusionist strategy can be considered a wish to be integrated into the establishment of the profession as a female mind doctor, these discussions demonstrate that she was successful.

We know from the details of Boyle's later career that she went on to become a major figure in the field and the responses to these early articles are evidence of her acceptance and the respect afforded her by male mind doctors. Indeed, in Boyle's obituary in the *British Medical Journal* in 1957, her colleagues speak most highly of her. Dr L. A. Parry in particular writes:

Her life showed so plainly how selfless she was: she lived for others. But she also enjoyed to the full her own life. She was a regular attendant at medical meetings, and seldom missed any of the social functions arranged by the various societies to which she belonged. And how she enjoyed them. She threw herself whole-heartedly into all that went on (C.L.H 1957, p. 1311).

This is the picture of a woman active and happy in her professional life, who had successfully integrated into mainstream psychiatry. This shift was not, of course, entirely due to Boyle's efforts but is reflective of wider changes in attitudes to medical women that had occurred in the early years of the twentieth century. Boyle's life included struggle and success as beliefs about women altered, in part due to the work which she and other female doctors like her undertook. Despite the difficulties she faced, Boyle was able to work within the constraints placed upon her by her sex, manipulating gendered ideologies to achieve her goals. Her biography shows how women were not merely passive recipients of these ideas but often active participants in their making as well as their deconstruction. For Boyle, this meant making use of textual practices within her discipline to pursue dual separatist and inclusionist strategies, ensuring that she was able to retain autonomy over her work at the same time as cultivating professional acceptance. Boyle's writing was an integral part of her professional practice and the texts she published made a significant contribution to the success of her career ambitions.

References

Unpublished Sources

Annual Reports of the Lewes Road Hospital and Lady Chichester Hospital and Dispensary. 1900–1914. London Archives. HB/18/1/63/1/1A.

Application Form 249: Helen Boyle. 1889. London School of Medicine for Women. London Archives. H72/SM/C/01/02/001.

Claybury Sub-Committee Minutes. 1874–1875. London Archives. LCC/MIN/00920.

Claybury Sub-Committee Minutes. 1875–1876. London Archives. LCC/MIN/00921.

Elston, Mary Ann C. 1986. Women Doctors in the British Health Services: A Sociological Study of their Careers and Opportunities. PhD thesis: University of Leeds. https://etheses.whiterose.ac.uk/247/. Accessed 31 December 2024.

Jex-Blake, Sophia. 1887. *Medical Women: A Ten Years' Retrospect*. London Archives. H72/SJB/01/002.

Lady Chichester Hospital Register of Patients. 1905–1910. London Archives. HB/80/1.

Lady Chichester Hospital Register of Patients. 1910–1914. London Archives. HB/80/2.

London School of Medicine for Women Prospectus. 1874–1897. London Archives. H72/SM/C/01/01/001.

London School of Medicine for Women Results of School Examinations. 1874–1900. H72/SM/C/01/04/001

Milliken, Emma. 2010. Treating Borderline Mental Illness in Twentieth-Century Britain: The Pioneering Contribution of Dr Helen Boyle, with Particular Reference to the Foundation of the Lady Chichester Hospital. PhD Thesis: University of Westminster. University of Westminster Archive. SOC:PHD Box no. 04373652.

Published Sources

A Clerical Correspondent. 1889. Women Physicians at Clapham. *Hospital*. 6: 403–403.

Anger, Suzy. 2009. *Journal of Mental Science* (1853-). In *Dictionary of Nineteenth-Century Journalism in Great Britain and Ireland*, ed. by Laurel Brake and Marysa Demoor, 325. Ghent: Academia Press.

Berrios, German E., and Hugh Freeman, ed. 1991. *150 Years of British Psychiatry, 1841–1991, Vol. I* London: Gaskell.

Blake, Catriona. 1990. *The Charge of the Parasols: Women's Entry to the Medical Profession*. New York: Women's Press.

Bourdillon, Hilary. 1988. *Women as Healers: A History of Women and Medicine*. Cambridge: Cambridge University Press.

Boyle, Helen. 1899. A Case of Juvenile General Paralysis. *Journal of Mental Science* 45: 99–105.

Boyle, Helen. 1905. Some Points in the Early Treatment of Mental and Nervous Cases (with Special Reference to the Poor). *Journal of Mental Science*. 51: 676–681.

Boyle, Helen. 1909. Account of an Attempt at the Early Treatment of Mental and Nervous Cases (with Special Reference to the Poor). *Journal of Mental Science*. 55: 683–692.

Boyle, Helen. 1914. Some Observations on Early and Nervous Mental Cases, with Suggestions as to Possible Improvements in our Methods of Dealing with Them. *Journal of Mental Science*. 60: 381–398.

Boyle, Helen. 1939. Watchman, What of the Night? *Journal of Mental Science*. 358: 858–870.

British Architect Special Correspondence. 1886. *British Architect*. 25: 247–248.

Brock, Claire. 2007. The *Lancet* and the Campaign Against Women Doctors. In *Amanda Mordavsky Caleb, 130–145*, ed. (Re)Creating Science in Nineteenth-Century Britain, 1860–1880. Newcastle: Cambridge Scholars Publishing.

Brown, Michael. 2011. *Performing Medicine: Medical Culture and Identity in Provincial England, c.1760–1850*. Manchester: Manchester University Press.

Buklijas, Tatjana. 2017. The Laboratory and the Asylum: Francis Walker Mott and the Pathological Laboratory at London County Council Lunatic Asylum, Claybury, Essex (1895–1916). *History of Psychiatry*. 28: 311–325.

Bynum, William F. 1994. *Science and the Practice of Medicine in the Nineteenth Century*. Cambridge: Cambridge University Press.

Clark, Michael J. 1981. The Rejection of Psychological Approaches to Mental Disorder in Late Nineteenth-Century British Psychiatry. In *Madhouses, Mad-Doctors, and Madmen: The Social History of Psychiatry in the Victorian Era*, ed. Andrew Scull, 271–312. Philadelphia: University of Pennsylvania Press.

C.L.H. 1957. Obituary: Helen Boyle, M.D. *British Medical Journal*. 2: 1310–1312.

Lazenby Craig, Barbara. 1991. The Role of Records and of Recordkeeping in the Development of the Modern Hospital in London, England, and Ontario, Canada, c.1890–1940. *Bulletin of the History of Medicine*. 65: 367–397.

Crowther, M. Anne., and Marguerite Dupree. 2007. *Medical Lives in the Age of Surgical Revolution*. Cambridge: Cambridge University Press.

Csiszar, Alex. 2018. *Authorship and the Politics of Knowledge in the Nineteenth Century*. Chicago: Chicago University Press.

Dawson, Gowan, Bernard Lightman, Sally Shuttleworth, and Jonathan R. Topham, eds. 2020. *Science Periodicals in Nineteenth-Century Britain: Constructing Scientific Communities*. Chicago: Chicago University Press.

Elston, Mary Ann C. 2001. 'Run by Women (mainly) for Women': Medical Women's Hospitals in Britain, 1866–1948. In *Women and Modern Medicine*, ed. by Lawrence Conrad and Anne Hardy, 73–107. Leiden: Brill.

Engstrom, Edward J. 2003. *Clinical Psychiatry in Imperial Germany: a History of Psychiatric Practice*. Ithaca: Cornell University Press.

Feigned Insanity. 1883. *Chambers's Journal*. 20: 657–659.

Garrett Anderson, Louisa. 2016. *Elizabeth Garrett Anderson, 1836–1917*. Cambridge: Cambridge University Press.

Hardy, Anne, and Lawrence Conrad, eds. 2001. *Women and Modern Medicine*. Amsterdam: Rodopi.

Heasman, Kathleen J. 1964. The Medical Mission and the Care of the Sick Poor in Nineteenth-Century England. *Historical Journal*. 7: 230–245. https://doi.org/10.1017/S0018246X00025449.

Hide, Louise. 2014. *Gender and Class in English Asylums, 1890–1914*. Basingstoke: Palgrave Macmillan.

Jackson, William L. 2012. 'The Collector Will Call': Controlling Philanthropy through the Annual Reports of the Royal Infirmary of Edinburgh, 1837–1856. *Accounting History Review*. 22: 47–72. https://doi.org/10.1080/21552851.2012.653132.

Levine, Philippa, and Alison Bashford. 2012. Introduction: Eugenics and the Modern World. In *The Oxford Handbook of the History of Eugenics*, ed. Alison Bashford and Philippa Levine, 2–24. Oxford: Oxford University Press.

Lorkowski, Jacek, and Mieczyslaw Pokorski. 2022. Medical Records: A Historical Narrative. *Biomedicines*, 10: 2594. https://doi.org/ https://doi.org/10.3390/biomedicines10102594

Mackenzie, Charlotte. 1983. Women and Psychiatric Professionalisation. In *The London Feminist History Group, 107–119*, ed. The Sexual Dynamics and of History: Men's Power, Women's Resistance, 1780–1914. London: Pluto Press.

Marks, Lara. 1992. Mothers, babies and hospitals: 'The London' and the Provision of Maternity Care in East London, 1870–1939. In *Women and Children First*. London: Routledge.

McIntyre, Neil. 2014. *How British Women Became Doctors: The Story of the Royal Free Hospital and Its Medical School*. Croydon: Wenrowave Press.

Millikien, Emma. 2006. Helen Boyle (1869–1957). In *Oxford Dictionary of National Biography*. https://doi.org/10.1093/ref:odnb/60889. Accessed 1 January 2025.

Moulds, Alison. 2021. *Medical Identities and Print Culture, 1830s–1910s*. Cham: Palgrave Macmillan.

Pick, Daniel. 1989. *Faces of Degeneration: A European Disorder, c. 1848–1918*. Cambridge: Cambridge University Press.

Renvoize, Edward. 1991. The Association of Medical Officers of Asylums and Hospitals for the Insane, the Medico-Psychological Association, and their Presidents. In *150 Years of British Psychiatry, 1841–1991*, vol. I, ed. German E. Berrios and Hugh Freeman, 29–78. London: Gaskell.

Richardson, Angelique. 2003. *Love and Eugenics in the Late Nineteenth Century: Rational Reproduction and the New Woman*. Oxford: Oxford University Press.

Risse, Guenter B., and Harley Warner. 1992. Reconstructing Clinical Activities: Patient Records in Medical History. *Social History of Medicine*. 5: 183–205. https://doi.org/10.1093/shm/5.2.183.

Roelcke, Volker, Paul J. Weindling, and Louise Westwood, eds. 2010. *International Relations in Psychiatry: Britain, Germany, and the United States to World War II*. Woodbridge: University of Rochester Press.

Saunders, Janet. 1988. Quarantining the Weak-Minded: Psychiatric Definitions of Degeneracy and the Late-Victorian Asylum. in *Anatomy of Madness: Essays in the History of Psychiatry, III*, ed. by W.F. Bynum, Roy Porter, and Michael Shepherd, 273–296. Abingdon: Routledge.

Sheperd, Michael. 1992. Psychiatric Journals and the Evolution of Psychological Medicine. *Psychological Medicine*. 22: 15–25. https://doi.org/10.1017/S0033291700032682.

Shorter, Edward. 1998. *A History of Psychiatry: From the Era of the Asylum to the Age of Prozac*. Hoboken: Wiley.

Shuttleworth, Sally, and Berris Charnley. 2016. Science Periodicals in the Nineteenth and Twenty-First Centuries. *Notes and Records*. 70: 297–304. https://doi.org/10.1098/rsnr.2016.0026.

Stanton, Patricia, and John Stanton. 2002. Corporate Annual Reports: Research Perspectives Used. *Accounting, Auditing, and Accountability Journal*. 15: 478–500. https://doi.org/10.1108/09513570210440568.

Takabayashi, Akinobu. 2017. Surviving the Lunacy Act of 1890: English Psychiatrists and Professional Development during the Early Twentieth Century. *Medical History*. 61: 246–269. https://doi.org/10.1017/mdh.2017.4.

Thomson, Matthew. 2012. Disability, Psychiatry, and Eugenics. In *The Oxford Handbook of the History of Eugenics*, ed. Alison Bashford and Philippa Levine, 116–133. Oxford: Oxford University Press.

Turner, Trevor. 1991. 'Not Worth Powder and Shot': The Public Profile of the Medico-Psychological Association, c. 1851–1914. In *150 Years of British Psychiatry, 1841–1991, Vol I.* ed. by German E. Berrios and Hugh Freeman, 3–16. London: Gaskell.

Wallis, Jennifer. 2017. *Investigating the Body in the Victorian Asylum: Doctors, Patients, and Practices*. Basingstoke: Palgrave Macmillan.

Weisz, George. 2003. The Emergence of Medical Specialization in the Nineteenth Century. *Bulletin of the History of Medicine*. 77: 536–574. https://doi.org/10.1353/bhm.2003.0150.

Westwood, Louise. 2001. A Quiet Revolution in Brighton: Dr Helen Boyle's Pioneering Approach to Mental Health Care, 1899–1939. *Social History of Medicine*. 14: 439–457. https://doi.org/10.1093/shm/14.3.439.

Westwood, Louise. 2006. Separatism and Exclusion: Women in Psychiatry, 1900–50. In *Mental Illness and Learning Disability Since 1850: Finding a Place for Mental Disorder in the United Kingdom*, ed. Pamela Dale and Joseph Melling, 91–111. Abingdon: Routledge.

Witz, Anne. 1992. *Professions and Patriarchy*. London: Routledge.

CHAPTER 6

Conclusion: Interventions in the Historiography of Victorian Psychiatry

Much of the historiography of nineteenth-century psychiatry has focused on the rise of the asylum and the transformation of mental health care into a medical specialty. Historians have identified a period of professionalisation in psychiatric practice which occurred from the mid-nineteenth to early-twentieth century and covers the decades between the establishment of the Lunacy Commission and passage of the 1845 Lunacy Act, and the First World War. They have tended to interpret this period as a time in which the discipline was struggling to assert itself in the medical marketplace and establish its legitimacy as a field. Scholars have therefore suggested that the theories and clinical practices which became dominant in psychiatry during this time were shaped more by the desire to obtain authority and longevity as a discipline, than by a real interest in understanding and curing mental disease.

The anti-psychiatry movement of the 1960s and 70s has formed the backdrop for much recent work on the history of psychiatry. This group included several historians and academics (including Michel Foucault (1999) and Thomas Szasz (1970)) who studied the birth of medical care for the insane to understand how the discipline, as they thought, had failed so spectacularly. Heather Murray has demonstrated that one of the key arguments these thinkers made was that the 'very concept of madness was socially constructed' and that social control was (and is) inherent

M. Chapman, *Writing Women's Madness, 1845–1914*, Palgrave Studies in Literature, Science and Medicine,
https://doi.org/10.1007/978-3-031-97092-4_6

in the psychiatric system (Murray 2014, p. 38). They viewed psychiatry as 'an attempt to medicalize eccentric [or transgressive] behaviour' (Murray 2014, p. 38). Foucault in particular argued that the confinement of lunatic patients in asylums served the purpose of controlling a deviant population. It is this approach to the history of psychiatry that has led to criticism of Victorian mind doctors as dominating and oppressive.

In the late twentieth century, several social historians offered a revision of the work done by the anti-psychiatrists and put forward varying theories as to the significance of social control in the foundation of psychiatry as a profession (McGovern 1986). Perhaps the most reactionary was Edward Shorter, who described the anti-psychiatry movement as a 'store chest of scholarly hobbyhorses' (Shorter 1998, p. 52) and argued that the rise in asylum populations resulted from the redistribution of care from the community and 'a genuine increase in the rate of mental illness' (Shorter 1998, p. 53). However, other historians—most notably Andrew Scull (1993)—have adhered much more closely to the social control model. Whilst rejecting the anti-psychiatrist's conception of mental illness as socially constructed, he agrees that the dominance of the asylum within nineteenth-century psychiatry is the direct result of segregationist attitudes to deviant populations imposed by an intellectual, bourgeois elite. Many of these analyses present Victorian mind doctors and their treatments as semi-skilled at best and abusive at worst.

However, Marlene Arieno's compelling analysis has opened space for thinking about the development of the psychiatric profession as part of a complex web of intellectual, historical, and social factors. She argues that the social control theory is 'stunningly refuted by statistical evidence' (Arieno 1989, p. 73) that 'the institutionalised very closely parallel the general population with regard to age, sex, and social class' (Arieno 1989, p. 15). Indeed, she argues that 'the medical profession was so disorganised until well past mid-century that it would have been impossible for the professionals to accomplish any coherent plotting' (Arieno 1989, p. 315). Instead, Arieno (1989) suggests that two interconnected factors led to the proliferation of asylums and the importance of the physician within these institutions, through which the profession of psychiatry developed. Firstly, she argues that the centralisation of government in the Victorian era meant that state run institutions were the most likely solution to the problem of the insane during this time. The second factor which Arieno identifies is the shift from a spiritual to a disease model of insanity, which this book has focused on. The rising authority of science and medicine as an epistemological system allowed medical practitioners to stake a claim in the treatment of lunacy and asylum superintendents were increasingly required to possess medical expertise to hold the position. This gradually resulted in the professionalisation of mental health care.

Arieno's hypothesis is important as it offers scope for an analysis of the mind sciences which recognises the interaction of science, society, and culture. This is particularly important when considering medical beliefs about the gendered mind. This book has engaged with the foundational work of twentieth-century feminist historians, who have explored the role of social control in the theory and treatment of female insanity, suggesting that psychiatry policed women's bodies and behaviour by diagnosing deviancy from social norms as madness. These scholars also saw the asylum system as an arm of the patriarchal state, designed to contain and control disruptive women. Chesler's work (2005), originally published in 1972, is a radical feminist vision of anti-psychiatry. Showalter's study (1987) makes claims about the intention of psychiatric professionals to control and coerce women's behaviour. Russell's explanatory model (1995) likewise relates the actions of the Victorian psychiatric community to a deliberate and concerted effort of the profession to gain power or prestige.

Recent scholarship on the history of psychiatry and gender in the nineteenth century has tended to refute and revise these earlier accounts. Such studies, such as that of Andrews and Digby (2004), have demonstrated that the experience of female patients in the asylum is a lot more nuanced than historians such as Showalter (1987) or Foucault (1999) have supposed. So-called post-revisionist studies of nineteenth-century institutions for the insane have argued that the phenomenon of female incarceration is incorrect, with asylum admissions by and large (as Arieno indicated) reflecting the gender balance in wider society. They have also further explored the feminist perspective by challenging assumptions about psychiatric diagnosis and treatment of women, rejecting the claims put forward by Chesler (2005), Ussher (2011), and Showalter (1987) that psychiatry was used to police female behaviour. Through research centred on institutional data, historians such as David Wright have demonstrated that 'decisions over confinement rested on a delicate negotiation between families, local medical practitioners and Poor Law officers' (Wright 2004, p. 152), thus refuting the supposed 'imposition of a new *psychiatric* order on social behaviour' (Wright 2004, p. 159). This work has served to counter the notion that more women in Victorian society were found mad, and that they were labelled as such because of deviant behaviour specific and exclusive to their gender.

Such scholarship has been admirable for its empirical focus on archival materials and for its balancing of gender with other social factors such as class, to give a more detailed picture of the treatment of women in psychiatric practice. However, the epidemiological leanings of such studies in their emphasis on the incidence of female insanity, has resulted in a reduced awareness of the belief systems which lay behind and worked alongside more practical decisions and their consequences, like the need to quiet a noisy patient to maintain order on a ward. The stories of female patients at Crichton Royal Institution (Chapter 4) shed light on some of these factors, demonstrating how methodological differences in professional practice (such as the CRI's moral management therapeutics) impacted the treatment of women in one nineteenth-century asylum as much, and often more than, doctors' gendered beliefs about the female brain. Approaches to female insanity in the asylum were therefore complex and multifaceted, and not nearly as black-and-white as earlier historians have supposed.

Despite this, this book has demonstrated that *ideas* about female madness—its aetiology and nosology, and its social meanings—*were* gendered. Theories of female madness were often based on two interconnected beliefs: that women had a preponderance towards insanity on account of their frailer nervous system and reproductive cycle; and that the causes of their illness were related to their bodies, even if they were first refracted through the lens of 'moral' (social) catalysts. These beliefs were products of a social ideology that aligned women with nature, childbearing and rearing, emotionality, purity/sexuality, economic dependence, moral guardianship, feeble intellect, and domesticity, and were part of a web of behaviours, social and educational restrictions, and legislation which served to rearticulate and reinforce these values. Ideas about female insanity are inseparable from this cultural context, but also from the developing professional, medical context of which they were a part.

The research on Crichton Royal Institution for this book, alongside other recent historical work, suggests that there appears to be a gap between what doctors thought about madwomen and what they did about them: between ideology and practice. This can perhaps be explained by the difference between what was theorised at the forefront of psychiatric medicine (by men such as Bucknill and Tuke) and what was practised daily by run-of-the-mill mind doctors with an unruly asylum population to manage and financial margins to observe. However, I suggest that this divide may be an artificial one, created by binary thinking which has unhelpfully led to interpretations of nineteenth-century female madness falling into two camps: as misogynistic and controlling, or not.

The work of Joan Busfield (1996) is helpful here in breaking down this binary. Busfield offers one of the most nuanced studies of the relationship between gender and mental illness. She develops and complicates the work of earlier feminist scholars by approaching their claims from a sociological perspective and by including patients of both sexes in her analysis. Her study examines 'the institutions themselves, including the concepts with which they operate, and which are embedded in their practice,' to argue that 'what counts as unreason is socially variable: changing over time and differing between societies' (Busfield 1996, p. 232). Busfield concludes that 'gender, like social class and ethnicity, shapes judgements of unreason, and, consequently, the way in which the boundaries of mental disorder are determined for men and women, both in relation to the construction of categories of mental disorder and the identification of individual cases' (Busfield 1996, p. 234). Clinical practice is inevitably shaped by many factors, the ideology of the society in which the doctor lived and worked being just one. In fact, it is a more accurate representation to say that gendered ideas about the female mind were an *influence* upon the things that Victorian mind doctors thought, said, and did throughout this period. Exposed to these ideas through a variety of discourses (not least written and published documents), doctors necessarily involved them in the decisions they made about treating patients. Nevertheless, these ideas were not always the most important factor in these decisions, and it was possible to act in a way which challenged them.

Helen Boyle's clinical practice is a good example of this. Many aspects of her approach to women's mental health care were progressive but her engagement with gendered ideas of the female mind was itself unconventional. In her diagnosis of an adolescent girl with general paralysis, detailed in an article for the *Journal of Mental Science*, she offers an alternative reading of gender-specific symptoms. Boyle does not initially deviate from the late-Victorian consensus on the role of female reproductive organs in mental disease. She notices how the patient 'never menstruated at all' (Boyle 1899, p. 100) until the final stages of her illness, at which point 'the first signs of catamenia were ushered in by a severe convulsive attack' (Boyle 1899, p. 103). The patient's first menstruation was initially followed by temporary relief from symptoms, but she then worsened and died. Boyle also suggests that the patient being pubescent, ovarian activity may have had a profound effect on the disease. Boyle combines what she knows about the physiology of the onset of menstruation at puberty with contemporary understanding of the nature of general paralysis to 'suggest that [...] constitutional taints [from the parents] modified the ovarian secretion so that toxaemia occurred, either owing to the altered secretion itself or some by-product of the altered nutrition' (Boyle 1899, p. 104). The patient's inability to menstruate caused her disease. The pathology of insanity was a major focus of psychiatric research in the last decades of the century (and Boyle participated in these experiments with Mott at Claybury). These ideas must have held as much influence for Boyle as biological theories of women's madness. Her analysis of the girl's case is a synthesis of the many ideas which she was exposed to, through which she was able to expand upon and develop the biological basis for female insanity.

Indeed, it is important not to view women as passive recipients of either ideology or psychiatry in the nineteenth century. Women actively participated in the making of ideas about the female mind, as well as decisions over mental health care (whether personal or professional). From Boyle to H.T., Sophia Jex-Blake, Elizabeth Garrett Anderson, and Eliza Orme, women from inside and outside the medical professions were involved in writing, treating, and discussing mental illness. Again, this story is complex. The female response to psychiatry was not always one of resistance and a fight against oppression. Dominant ideologies are internalised and often reproduced even by those most negatively impacted by them. Some of these women continued to work within the limitations set by the Victorian concept of the female mind, even as they tried to create change for themselves and others. These nuances are often overlooked in twentieth-century feminist studies of Victorian attitudes to female madness and are rarely the focus of post-revisionist accounts of asylum statistics. Phyllis Chesler, for example, argues that 'most women in asylums were not insane' (Chesler 2005, p. 62), and that those—like Catherine Beecher and Charlotte Perkins Gilman—that 'believed that something really was wrong with them' mistakenly assigned their 'overwhelming fatigue and depression' to illness, rather than to an unconscious protest against their 'traditional "feminine" work—or overwork' (Chesler 2005, p. 69). This blanket application of her own ideological aims over the real feelings of her subjects clearly suppresses the voices of the women Chesler claims to defend. The work of Andrews and Digby (2004),

Wright (2004), and Shepard (2004), whilst significantly more balanced than Chesler's radical feminism, deals with the broad picture of institutional admissions and diagnostic patterns, and tells us little about the stories of individual women.

The historiography of nineteenth-century psychiatry is fraught and often politicised. Critical approaches to mental health care during the Victorian period have been shaped by shifting contemporary concerns about psychiatric treatment, so much so that the anti-psychiatrists and feminist critics that followed them now seem a piece of history of themselves. As Heather Murray (2014) has shown, historians of the 1960s through the 1980s were writing in a climate of antagonism between the psychiatric profession and lay people, particularly in the United States. She suggests that the origins of these historians' theories lay in their radical fears about hegemonic oppression in mid-twentieth-century Western society. They felt repressed by the clinical approaches prevalent in the 'social sciences characteristic of American modernity,' which they believed to suppress intuition, feeling and sensitivity (Murray 2014, p. 38). Murray argues that writers such as Foucault (1999) and Szasz (1970) conflated historical events with their own emotional reactions to modern psychiatry, creating a continuum of brutality between Victorian treatments and present-day medicine, the sole aim of which was to suppress social deviance. The work of Showalter (1987) and Ussher (2011), understood in this way, views psychiatry as an oppressive form of patriarchal control.

Scholarship published in the twenty-first century is the product of a different set of attitudes and a historiographical focus on the social causes of insanity reflects this. Some of the stigma around mental illness and the seeking of medical care has been overcome and fears over the nature and intention of this care have been allayed. In the last ten years, the problems of contemporary psychiatry have been posed in terms of funding and resources. In the United Kingdom, there are complaints about long waiting lists, patients slipping through the net, and the lack of NHS funding for mental health clinics and research. There is a call for greater access to treatment for more people. According to the 2016 Mental Health Taskforce's Five Year Forward View for Mental Health, 'too many people have received no help at all, leading to hundreds of thousands of lives put on hold or ruined, and thousands of tragic and unnecessary deaths' (NHS England 2016). The Forward View outlined planned improvements to be made in NHS mental health care and gave prevention, increased availability of care, an integrated approach to mental and physical health, and an end to underfunding as its key goals. The Forward View also recognised and sought to address the social causes and consequences of mental illness, such as poor housing, unemployment, addiction, crime, and lack of access to medical assistance. This led to a white paper in 2021 and the drafting of a reform bill for the Mental Health Act in 2022. Likewise, a 2021 spending review recommended investment to ensure patients can access mental health services in a timely fashion, to keep as well as possible.

Across all these studies, there has been a need to prove whether the Victorians treated the insane badly, and whether this was intentional (this has particularly been the case with female patients). The creation of psychiatry as a medical discipline feels personal. Perhaps this emotive engagement with the past is because the evolution of the field in Western medicine can be traced directly to the work of these nineteenth-century mind doctors and the concurrent decline in the spiritual concept of the mind. In the UK, our use of medical services for mental health results from the relatively recent changes in law and clinical practice heralded by the Lunacy Act of 1845 and Lunacy (Scotland) Act of 1857. There is, too, a thread of commonality between the late-Victorian mind sciences and the methods used in twentieth and twenty-first-century psychiatry. The development of medical institutions for the mentally ill, drug treatments, psychological therapies, and the clinical and pathological focus on the brain all began during the first decades of professional psychiatry and remain the hallmarks of the field today. Indeed, Busfield includes the history of nineteenth-century psychiatry in her work only because 'twentieth-century ideas manifest the types of biologism and gender bias' of the earlier era (Busfield 1996, p. 9). 'As in the nineteenth-century, much of the emphasis in explaining the gendered landscape is on reproductive differences between men and women,' though focus is now on 'genetically based hormonal differences,' rather than the obscure mechanical influence of the womb on the nerves (Busfield 1996, p. 154).

Significantly, this book has shown how nineteenth-century ideas about the female mind were communicated in writing, which was of enormous importance to the professional practice of psychiatry during this period. Texts written and read both from within and outside the primary sites of practice in the mind sciences had the ability to influence what practicing doctors thought. The texts themselves took on an active role in shaping psychiatric theories through their use and consumption by mind doctors, other medical professionals, and lay members of the public. The constraints of genre, audience and form shaped the content published, determining what was communicated. Writing thus had a fundamental impact on thinking about female insanity, as well as other forms of mental disorder.

Many of the textual discourses which developed during the Victorian period remain the backbone of communication and education within the profession today. The *Journal of Mental Science* became the *British Journal of Psychiatry* in 1963, the MPA itself evolving into the Royal College of Psychiatrists in 1971. The *BJP* is still one of the major publications in the field, describing itself as 'a leading international peer-reviewed journal, covering all branches of psychiatry with a particular emphasis on the clinical aspects of each topic' (Royal College of Psychiatrists 2024). It is 'committed to improving the prevention, investigation, diagnosis, treatment, and care of mental illness' (Royal College of Psychiatrists 2024). Much like its Victorian iteration, the journal is a tool for the promotion of the discipline and the communication of research amongst colleagues (Fyfe et al. 2015; Topham 2014; Dawson et al. 2020). The periodical is the accepted (and expected) genre for scholarly and professional publications across many disciplines. The 'modern scientific journal,' as Alex Csiszar has shown, 'is largely an invention of the nineteenth century' (Csiszar 2018, p. 4). Over the hundred years or so following the French Revolution, 'scientific practitioners began to perceive the existence of a single, cohesive-enough genre—the scientific paper—as the chief avenue by which to make the results of their research into public knowledge claims' (Csiszar 2018, p. 4). During this period, 'specialised serials came to form the solid core of science in print,' at the same time as the scientific author became an identifiable discrete personage (Csiszar 2018, p. 8). By the end of the nineteenth century, 'it was widely acknowledged that a career and reputation in science depended largely on one's unpaid contributions to particular kinds of periodicals' (Csiszar 2018, p. 9). This is a trend which, Csiszar argues, has continued into our own age.

The psychiatric textbook is likewise a genre still used in the standardisation of knowledge and as an educational tool for practitioners and students alike. The *Diagnostic and Statistical Manual*, produced by the American Psychiatric Association and in its 5th edition, is a reference bible accessible to medical professionals of all kinds. It is intended as a tool to aid in diagnosis, giving currently accepted classifications of disorders organised by the symptoms they present. Whilst the *DSM-V* has been much criticised for the relationship between the pharmaceutical industry and its revision taskforce, and for the lack of empirical evidence it provides, it remains a cornerstone text of the discipline (particularly for US practitioners; in the UK the World Health Organisation's *International Classification of Diseases* is more commonly used). There is still a need for a guide to help doctors make sense of an uncertain field, to navigate clinical decisions without personal expertise. One of the disciplinary building activities of the Royal College of Psychiatrists is to campaign for better training in psychiatry, both to ensure that all health professionals can recognise and diagnose mental illness, and so that those medical students interested in a career in psychiatry can progress with the necessary skills. In September 2019, the College published guidance on the implementation of psychiatric education following the 2018 General Medical Council policy on graduate outcomes, in which it was recommended that all medical graduates should understand the 'principles for the identification, safe management and referral of patients with mental health conditions' (General Medical Council 2018). In its guidance, the College asserted that 'having insufficient professionals able to treat people with mental illness is now widely recognised as one of the biggest risks to achieving parity of esteem between mental and physical health' (Royal College of Psychiatrists 2019). The problem of education, and the tools to combat this, are remarkably similar to the concerns expressed by Victorian mind doctors.

These connections have made the study of nineteenth-century psychiatry a study of practices which affect individuals in the present. The experiences of Victorian patients, too, feel remarkably close to home when the treatments and diagnoses patients receive today are reminiscent of those used in the period. Research into the history of the field, and particularly its relationship to marginalised groups, is important to better understand how these practices arose and can be improved. Nevertheless, it is ahistorical (and overly simplistic) to pass judgement on nineteenth-century physicians, policy makers, and the psychiatric profession as a whole. With this book I have tried to recognise and unpack the social and textual structures through which beliefs about the female mind were formed. Psychiatry, in the past and present, should be viewed (like all science and medicine) as part of a social and cultural network of ideas, not as a discrete and pure dispenser of ultimate truth, nor a malignant set of practices implemented by a group of individuals with designs on power. Approaching the history of psychiatry with an understanding of the conditions in which knowledge claims are made will better our ability to situate both historical and contemporary medical treatments within the wide context which influences their development.

References

Published Sources

Andrews, Jonathan, and Anne Digby, eds. 2004. *Sex and Seclusion, Class and Custody: Perspectives on Gender and Class in the History of British and Irish Psychiatry*. New York: Rodopi.

Arieno, Marlene A. 1989. *Victorian Lunatics: A Social Epidemiology of Mental Illness in Mid-Nineteenth-Century England*. London: Associated University Presses.

Boyle, Helen. 1899. A Case of Juvenile General Paralysis. *Journal of Mental Science*. 45: 99–105.

Busfield, Joan. 1996. *Men, Women and Madness: Understanding Gender and Mental Disorder*. Basingstoke: Macmillan Press.

Chesler, Phyllis. 2005. *Women and Madness*. Rev. New York: Palgrave Macmillan.

Csiszar, Alex. 2018. *Authorship and the Politics of Knowledge in the Nineteenth Century*. Chicago: Chicago University Press.

Dawson, Gowan, Bernard Lightman, Sally Shuttleworth, and Jonathan R. Topham, eds. 2020. *Science Periodicals in Nineteenth-Century Britain: Constructing Scientific Communities*. Chicago: Chicago University Press.

Foucault, Michel. 1999. *Madness and Civilisation: A History of Insanity in the Age of Reason*, trans. by Richard Howard. London: Routledge.

Fyfe, Aileen, Julie McDougall-Waters, and Noah Moxam. 2015. 350 Years of Scientific Periodicals. *Notes and Records*. 69: 227–239. https://doi.org/10.1098/rsnr.2015.0036.

General Medical Council. 2018. *Outcomes for Graduates 2018*. https://www.gmc-uk.org/-/media/documents/dc11326-outcomes-for-graduates-2018_pdf-75040796.pdf. Accessed 30 December 2024.

McGovern, Constance M. 1986. Myths of Social Control and Custodial Oppression: Patterns of Psychiatric Medicine in Late Nineteenth-Century Institutions. *Journal of Social History*. 20: 3–23. https://doi.org/10.1353/jsh/20.1.3.

Murray, Heather. 2014. 'My Place Was Set At The Terrible Feast': The Meanings of the 'Anti-Psychiatry' Movement and Responses in the United States, 1970s–1990s. *Journal of American Culture*. 37: 37–51. https://doi.org/10.1111/jacc.12105.

NHS England. 2016. *The Five Year Forward View for Mental Health*, a report from the independent Mental Health Taskforce to the NHS in

England. https://www.england.nhs.uk/wp-content/uploads/2016/02/Mental-Health-Taskforce-FYFV-final.pdf. Accessed 30 December 2024.

Royal College of Psychiatrists. 2019. *Choose Psychiatry: Guidance for Medical Schools*. https://www.rcpsych.ac.uk/docs/default-source/become-a-psychiatrist/guidance-for-medical-schools-pdf.pdf?sfvrsn=20f46cae_14. Accessed 30 December 2024.

Royal College of Psychiatrists. 2024. *The Royal College of Psychiatrists (1971-): The History of the Royal College of Psychiatrists*, https://www.rcpsych.ac.uk/about-us/library-and-archives/our-history/the-rcpsych. Accessed 30 December 2024.

Scull, Andrew. 1993. *The Most Solitary of Afflictions: Madness and Society in Britain, 1700–1900*. New Haven: Yale University Press.

Shepard, Anne. 2004. The Female Patient Experience in Two Late-Nineteenth-Century Surrey Asylums. In *Sex and Seclusion, Class and Custody*, ed. Jonathan Andrews and Anne Digby, 223–248. New York: Rodopi.

Shorter, Edward. 1998. *A History of Psychiatry: From the Era of the Asylum to the Age of Prozac*. Hoboken: Wiley.

Showalter, Elaine. 1987. *The Female Malady: Women, Madness, and English Culture, 1830–1980*. London: Virago.

Szasz, Thomas S. 1970. *The Manufacture of Madness: A Comparative Study of the Inquisition and the Mental Health Movement*. New York: Harper and Row.

Topham, Jonathan R. 2013. Anthologizing the Book of Nature: the Circulation of Knowledge and the Origins of the Scientific Journal in Late Georgian Britain. In *The Circulation of Knowledge between Britain, India, and China: The Early-Modern World to the Twentieth Century*, ed. by Bernard Lightman et al., 119–152. Boston: Brill.

Ussher, Jane M. 2011. *The Madness of Women: Myth and Experience*. Hove: Routledge.

Wright, David. 2004. Delusions of Gender?: Lay Identification and Clinical Diagnosis of Insanity in Victorian England. In *Sex and Seclusion, Class and Custody*, ed. Jonathan Andrews and Anne Digby, 149–176. New York: Rodopi.

Index

M. Chapman, *Writing Women's Madness, 1845–1914*, Palgrave Studies in Literature, Science and Medicine,
https://doi.org/10.1007/978-3-031-97092-4

The manufacturer's authorised representative in the EU is Springer Nature Customer Service Centre GmbH, Europaplatz 3, 69115 Heidelberg, Germany. If you have any concerns regarding our products, please contact ProductSafety@springernature.com

Printed and bound by CPI Group (UK) Ltd, Croydon, CR0 4YY
05/10/2026
02228125-0002